D1071984

Coordinated Service Delivery Systems for the Elderly

*New Approaches
for Care and Referral
in New York State*

The *Advanced Models and Practice in Aged Care* series:

Number 1

The Acting-Out Elderly edited by Miriam K. Aronson, Ruth Bennett, and Barry J. Gurland

Number 2

Coordinated Service Delivery Systems for the Elderly: New Approaches for Care and Referral in New York State edited by Ruth Bennett, Susana Frisch, Barry J. Gurland, and David Wilder

Number 3

Aging & Communication: Problems in Management edited by Carol N. Wilder and Barbara E. Weinstein

Series Editors: Ruth Bennett, PhD, and Barry J. Gurland, MD, MRCP

Advanced Models and Practice in Aged Care
Number 2

Coordinated Service Delivery Systems for the Elderly

New Approaches for Care and Referral in New York State

Edited by

Ruth Bennett, PhD
Susana Frisch, MA
Barry J. Gurland, MD, MRCP
David Wilder, PhD

Center for Geriatrics and Gerontology
Columbia University

*HV
1468
·N7
C66
1984*

229323

The Haworth Press
New York

The Haworth Press, Inc., 28 East 22 Street, New York, NY 10010

Library of Congress Cataloging in Publication Data
Main entry under title:

Coordinated service delivery systems for the elderly.

(Advanced models and practice in aged care ; no. 2)
Bibliography: p.
1. Aged—Services for—New York (State)—Addresses, essays, lectures. 2. Community health services for the aged—New York (State)—Addresses, essays, lectures. 3. Long term care of the sick—New York (State)—Addresses, essays, lectures. I. Bennett, Ruth, 1933- . II. Series. [DNLM: 1. Health services for the aged—Organization and administration—New York—Congresses. 2. Community health services—Organization and administration—New York—Congresses. 3. Health planning—Organization and administration—New York—Congresses. 4. Long term care—Congresses. WT 30 C7778 1981]
HV1468.N7C66   1983   362.1'6'0973   83-13041
ISBN 0-86656-157-9

CONTENTS

PART III

KEY ISSUES

PART IV

CONCLUSIONS

APPENDICES

Acknowledgments

The Conference on Coordinated Service Delivery Systems in Long Term Care: The State of the Art in the State of New York was the result of several months of planning and coordination efforts with valuable input from the representatives of the co-sponsoring agencies. Their commitment to the success of the conference was evidenced by their active participation in the planning process and generous contribution of their time devoted to the production of papers included in this volume. Special thanks are also extended to Gerta Gruen for her assistance in recording and to Margaret Diaz, Debbie King, and Mari Schatz for their help in transcribing tapes and manuscripts.

*   *   *

This volume contains the proceedings of the conference on Coordinated Service Delivery Systems for Long Term Care: The State of the Art in the State of New York, held October 6 and 7, 1981 at the Alumni Auditorium of the College of Physicians and Surgeons, 630 West 168th Street, New York, New York. The conference was sponsored by the Center for Geriatrics and Gerontology and Long Term Care Gerontology Center, Columbia University Faculty of Medicine and New York State Office of Mental Health. Co-sponsors included the following: New York State Office for the Aging, New York City Department for the Aging, Columbia University Brookdale Institute on Aging and Adult Human Development, Fordham University Third Age Center, Jamaica Service Program for Older Adults, Metropolitan Jewish Geriatric Center, Albert Einstein College of Medicine, and Monroe County Long Term Care Program. The conference coordinator was Susana Frisch.

Preface

The community-based coordinated service system for the delivery of long-term care is a bold, new concept. To examine the broad array of relevant issues and problems, a conference was convened by the Columbia University Center for Geriatrics and Gerontology in October 1981. Co-sponsored by eight other New York State organizations and attended by numerous representatives from universities, service agencies, and other interested persons, the conference provided a forum for exchange of information on the operation, management, costs, and evaluation of such systems. It brought together many of the organizations currently conducting coordinated service delivery programs in several communities of New York State, and it was felt that such innovative programs need to be brought to the attention of the larger community, a process requiring both a conference and the wide circulation of proceedings.

This volume contains mostly the presentations made during the conference as well as discussions and concluding remarks. The emphasis is not only on the state of the art but also on the art in the State.

Papers in this volume contain descriptions of programs in Albany, Buffalo, New York City, Troy, and Rochester—all cities in the State of New York. New York State potentially has one of the largest and most complex health and social service systems in the world. New York State has seen the initiation of many innovations in health and social care. These pioneering efforts have made important contributions to raising the quality of care for the elderly both in New York and in the nation. Efforts are continuing and this conference and resulting proceedings are meant to serve as a showcase for these accomplishments, to help maintain a strong sense of identity for all of us in the field of long-term care, and to share with others the creative energies of those involved.

The impetus for the development of community-based coordinated service systems of long-term care seems to have come in part from a fiscal imperative and in part from a social or, perhaps, moral imperative. The fiscal imperative relates to the idea that provision of coordinated services in the community will prevent institutionalization and, therefore, be less costly; the social-moral imperative relates to the notion of providing services in the least restrictive setting in order to normalize the lives of the elderly as much as possible.

"Normalization" as a national long-term care policy goal was pioneered in Sweden. (Swedish aging policy was described at a seminar entitled "Facing an Aging Society" held at the Swedish Consulate in New York City, October 1978.)

In the United States, the National Long Term Care Demonstration Program was begun by the Department of Health and Human Services in 1979 to explore alternative approaches to community-based, long-term care in a systematic fashion and in so doing to determine: which approaches to organizing and delivering long-term care services have the greatest potential for achieving particular policy objectives; what the barriers to their implementation might be; and what their cost implications are.* Perhaps, after data are in from some of the projects described in this volume, community-based, long-term care will become national policy in this country as well.

DEFINITIONS

By community-based coordinated service systems for the delivery of long-term care, we mean the skillful packaging, timing, and monitoring of medical, nursing, social, personal, and other services delivered in the community to those in need of long-term care. "Channeling"—mentioned in several of the following chapters—refers to a case management approach to organizing and delivering community-based health and social services to chronically impaired persons. After screening and assessment, clients are linked via case management with community services appropriate to their needs. The Channeling Demonstration Program (funded under the National Long Term Care Demonstration) is a research program designed to test the effectiveness and efficiency of this approach to organizing and delivering services and controlling costs.

---

*See Unpublished Report for the evaluation of the National Long Term Care Demonstration by Mathematica Policy Research Inc., Princeton, N.J.

MODELS OF PRACTICE

One aspect of coordinated services is the professionalization of personal care. By that is meant that service packages are tailor-made for target groups or individuals who can benefit from them. Some of the projects described in this volume illustrate how this is done. Usually the notion of case management is a guiding principle for the delivery of coordinated services, and this is discussed in some detail in this volume.

A variety of service models have emerged. In some organizations, each package of services is put together by a nurse and a social worker who serve as case managers and who "prescribe" services based on extensive assessment. Usually, they do not deliver services; their job is to package them and to monitor their delivery. In some communities, attempts are made to fill service gaps when a particular service is needed but is not readily available. While the actual service delivery may not require a great amount of skill, e.g., meal or housekeeping service delivery, the packaging, timing, and targeting certainly do require skill. Formal training in case management skills has yet to be sufficiently operationalized so that trained case managers would be available to direct community programs.

A case* example based on the efforts of the Triage Project, a community-based coordinated service system in the State of Connecticut may serve as an illustration of how services are packaged and coordinated.

Mrs. H., at 92 years of age, was a severely disabled woman who lived alone in elderly housing. Her sight had failed, so that she could only see shapes, and, due to advanced osteoarthritis, she was unsteady when ambulating with her walker. Mrs. H. knew where everything was in her cluttered apartment as long as some well-meaning home care provider "didn't clean up." It was not unusual for Mrs. H. to spend one night a month on the floor, having fallen after getting up in the middle of the night to go to the bathroom. She had experienced the alternative: being tied in a chair for three weeks in a skilled nursing facility because the staff feared she might fall. To Mrs. H., that arrangement was totally unacceptable.

As the result of the assessment and coordination process, Mrs. H.

---

*The case of Mrs. H. was presented by Jane Birk of Triage at the National Association of State Units on Aging and National Area Agency Association meetings in Washington, D.C., July 26-28, 1981.

was able to return to her home. To maintain her at home, Triage co-ordinated the following services: a home health aide, one hour a day, from 8 to 9 a.m., from a non-profit agency; three hours a day, from 5 to 8 p.m., from a proprietary agency; home delivered meals every day at noon; and a monthly nursing visit to pour her medi-cation into individual envelopes. Even if Mrs. H. had a problem and Triage could not check on her, the coordinated care plan prevented her from going more than several hours without assistance. With Triage's help, she was able to enjoy independent living in her own home for the next four years.

SPECIAL ISSUES

Perhaps the case described above makes the effort required by co-ordination of services seem expensive. The issue of how to pay for coordination of services is very important and will be addressed in this volume. But cost may not be the critical issue to be faced. Orga-nization/coordination may be a crucial issue because it is well known that there are many reasons to prevent agencies from co-ordinating their efforts; e.g., different eligibility criteria, geo-graphic limitations, and turf battles. The issue of organization, especially as it relates to coordination, will also be addressed in this volume. Another crucial issue is determination of effectiveness: does the program work and how do we know it? The issues of eval-uation and assessment are addressed in this volume as well.

If community-based coordinated service programs can be demon-strated to work effectively, that is, improve significantly the quality of lives of the elderly and other long-term care consumers and their families and if the fact of their effectiveness is publicized, the public will demand the types of program packages developed by commu-nity-based coordinated service systems. At that point, the cost issue will surface seriously and, undoubtedly, will be resolved.

INFORMATION DISSEMINATION

A word or two, a digression perhaps, about the importance and modes of diffusion of information on innovations. If a bold new ef-fort such as the organization of community-based service delivery systems is to succeed, the information diffusion process needs to be speeded up. Especially in a period of scarce resources, when new programs are likely to be prematurely terminated, not because they are inefficient or ineffective but because they are not given a chance to prove themselves, frequent exchange of information on results is vital.

Information diffusion about innovations in the human service arena seems to follow several patterns:

1. Slow, trial-and-error diffusion: In the past, innovation in the human service arena seemed to require a lengthy process, at least in some fields. For example, it took about 50 years for the idea of kindergarten to be adopted throughout the educational system in the U.S., occurring through a slow process of tinkering and trial and error.

2. Change agent diffusion: Post World War II saw a speeding up of educational and other human service innovations largely through the support of foundations and governmental agencies. These agencies supported change agents, i.e., those local leaders who spread the word about innovations developed by "risk takers." Both the Agricultural Extension Services and the Office of Education adopted models of change agents who were supported for the explicit purpose of helping to grease the wheels of the diffusion and adoption processes. This process, too, allowed for tinkering, trial, and error.

3. Truncated diffusion: In the 1960s we began to confront a new model of diffusion in the human service arena with which we still seem to be saddled. At the time of the Great Society, truncated or instant diffusion seemed to be the order of the day. This instant diffusion seemed to take two forms: mandated diffusion and contest diffusion. In mandated diffusion, it was expected of a local community to adopt whatever new service was federally mandated; in contest diffusion, RFPs were circulated and the hopeful innovators competed with each other for funds to start a program in a local community. Under these conditions there was little time for tinkering and trial and error. Under conditions of truncated diffusion, several similar service programs were started up simultaneously in a number of different sites without the benefit derived from the slow trial and error process.

Today, many of our service programs find that they have been started up in this manner. With the truncating of the developmental and evolutionary diffusion processes, the expertise that grows out of tinkering and trial and error is not available. As a result, a knowledge vacuum develops and programs run the risk of failing due to lack of expertise. Thus, today, there is a great need for people who are involved in the same sort of human service work to get together, to share problems, and to learn from one another. They should even be able to respond collectively in order to reduce their pluralistic ignorance about demands placed upon them by sponsors or funding agencies. Perhaps this continual exchange of information about innovation could prevent some of the outcomes found in our studies of innovative programs in long-term care institutions (Bennett, R., and Wilder, D., 1980), namely that when the funding stopped, the programs stopped even though they were effective.

It is hoped community-based coordinated service delivery systems are not poised on the brink of such an occurrence. At the present time, when funds are being reduced therefore requiring a greater effort at coordination of scarce services, it would be ironic indeed for such systems to fail for lack of support. At this time, it probably is important to protect and expand the community-based coordinated service delivery systems which have just begun to be operational and to widely disseminate information about their experiences and results.

This conference and the present volume based on the conference proceedings are viewed not as the last but as the first word in an ongoing dialogue involving providers, consumers, and researchers in the long-term care field.* For the future, follow-up meetings are planned in order to cover in depth some of the issues and special problems described in these proceedings. In our view, exchange and diffusion of information on innovative programs is crucial for their improvement and perhaps survival.

ORGANIZATION OF VOLUME

This volume is organized as follows:

Part I contains papers on long-term care policy issues nationally and in New York State;

---

*This conference followed a similar conference held in Albany in June 1981, the proceedings of which were not published.

Part II contains descriptions of several community-based coordinated service programs in New York State;

Part III consists of discussions of four key issues in this field:
(1) systems organization, utilization, access, and gatekeeping
(2) case management
(3) costs and benefits
(4) assessment/evaluation;

Part IV contains concluding remarks and suggested issues for further discussion.

Appendices include recommended readings and a list of conference participants.

Part I

LONG-TERM CARE POLICY ISSUES NATIONALLY AND IN NEW YORK STATE

Introduction to Part I

Part I contains three papers:

- The first, by Monsignor Charles Fahey, deals with long-term care policy issues nationally, in light of changing demographics of the older population, changing values and ethics underlying federal and state policy considerations, and changing structures within formal and informal support systems;
- The second, by Robert O'Connell, describes the need for New York State to develop a statewide long-term care plan, providing its historical background as well as describing the initial stages of the planning effort and its administrative components;
- The third paper, by Marilyn Pickett-Desmond, describes nine policy options which illustrate different scenarios and issues that are being considered within the framework of the statewide plan development process.

National Perspective
on Issues of Long-Term Care

Monsignor Charles J. Fahey

The long-term care system serves those persons who will not fit somewhere else yet whose hurts so bother our collective conscience that we must do something.

This overview of issues in the field will have six main parts with several subunits. It is presented in this manner so that leaders in the field might use it as a framework for discussion:

1. Population at Risk
   a. demographics
   b. health status
   c. informal supports
   d. utilization patterns
2. Federal Policy
   a. resource transfers
   b. system building
   c. planning
   d. regulation
3. State Policy
   a. resource allocation
   b. locus of decision making
4. Local Issues
   a. system and function
   b. planning and administration
5. Non-Governmental
   a. sponsorship
   b. private investment
   c. private philanthropy
   d. trade organizations

Monsignor Charles J. Fahey is Director, Third Age Center, Fordham University, New York, N.Y.

6. Societal Values
   a. personal responsibility
   b. family roles
   c. social insurance
   d. welfare
   e. quality of life

1. Population at Risk

a. Demographics

The Federal Council on Aging recently released a study entitled, *The Need for Long Term Care.* It utilizes a number of studies to give some hint of future need. Were a number of variables held constant, expenditures for nursing home care would rise from $16 billion in 1978 to $76 billion in 1990. The number of nursing home beds would increase from 1,341,000 in 1978 to 1,997,000 in the year 2000.[1]

While it is unlikely that the expenditures in 1990 will be any less, it is equally unlikely that we will have a 50% increase in beds by the year 2000. However, these figures give some indication as to the crisis we face.

Persons have been defined out of acute care hospitals as well as out of state mental institutions. The nursing home is the final resource for those whose disabilities and hurts defy remedy by definition. Despite rapid increase, long-term care services, both in-patient and out, have kept pace with demand only because they too have defined clients so that only those who are the sickest and most distressed find their way into the system.

b. Health Status

Dr. James Fries, in his celebrated article in the *New England Journal of Medicine*,[2] identified the squaring of the survival curve. We can expect that 2/3 of Americans will live into their eighties. If we add three years in either direction to this decade, i.e., 77-93, we can expect 90% will live to within this age framework.

It is not certain what the decrease in mortality rate at earlier years means to the disability rate of the old, old. He describes a positive scenario based on better therapeutic intervention in the area of heart, stroke, and cancer.

Others of us feel that degenerative organic brain disease may occasion the need for more long-term care since its incidence rises with age.

It is impossible to assess such factors as women working and change in public policy in regard to public health and environmental control.

However, it is likely we will experience more chronicity rather than less. Of special note is the vulnerability of women. The longevity of women (they live on the average seven years longer than men) makes them particularly at risk. The large majority of persons in formal long-term care settings are women.

c. Informal Supports

While a "soft figure," it is estimated that 75% of persons with disabilities are cared for within the context of family, friends, neighbors—outside formal systems of care.

Despite a number of structural (e.g., size of houses) and cultural (e.g., movement of people) obstacles, informal care continues to be extraordinarily important. Only now are policy makers examining the impact of public policy and professional programs on the ecology of human interactions around frailty.

What of the future? On the positive side, the number of older women who are childless is at its peak (because of low fertility during the Depression period). On the other hand, the normalcy of four and five generations as well as the increased number of divorces portend problems. While 15% of men over 65 live alone, nearly 41% of women over 65 are so situated. "Living alone" is a major factor in "at riskness."[3]

It appears that the dominant factor in the informal support system is the long time interaction of people rather than any short-term public or professional intervention. If people laughed together over the years, they are likely to care for one another in tears.

The area of informal supports deserves our careful and respectful study.

d. Utilization Patterns

It is only when we look at care systems as a whole that we gain perspective on need. Hospitals, mental health facilities, and nursing homes interact with one another just as they do with both social and home health care services.

Today's patterns of care have been influenced largely by funding patterns. They are an illustration of the Sutton principle at work. When asked why he robbed banks, Willie Sutton is reported to have said: "because that is where the money is."

State government's first principle has been to maximize Medicare (no state money being involved). The second has been to maximize Medicaid (open-ended federal matching funding). Virtually every human frailty has been defined as a medical problem to capture federal Medicaid funds. It is questionable whether this policy has resulted in the most humane and economic technique of meeting human need.

2. *Federal Policy*

a. *Resource Transfers*

Since the Roosevelt Administration, the federal government has played an active role in a variety of societal activities and relationships. It has been concerned with the transfer of resources to the "have nots" even as it has concerned itself with access to service, non-discrimination, quality of care, and other humanitarian considerations.

It has assumed a social insurance as well as welfare function. Both are premised on the conviction that life, liberty, and pursuit of happiness imply that persons are entitled to food, clothing, shelter, and medical care. If the market place mechanism is unable to guarantee these, the government, at the federal level as well as the local level, has a responsibility to individual citizens. We have enacted several entitlement programs such as Medicare, Medicaid, and supplemental security insurance. They are the basic fabric of our Long-Term Care system.

The Reagan Administration has articulated a position which not only addresses the fiscal problems associated with frailty but also calls into question the philosophy underguarding the entitlement approach.

The Administration's position is that government should stay out of the market place and allow its forces to develop strong and vibrant economy from which all will benefit.

b. *System Building*

This philosophy of government in general and the federal government in particular challenges the common wisdom prevailing both in the public and private sectors for the past 20 years. Nonetheless, whether it be in the name of better access or effective economics, the private and public sectors seem committed to the development of health systems at the local level.

Even such trade organizations as the American Hospital Association, the American Medical Association, and the American Association of Homes for the Aging have encouraged their constituents to develop systems, albeit voluntary, back in "River City."

The Reagan Administration, to the applause of some actors in the field, calls for a radical change in approach even as it has in the overall economic system of the nation. Let the market place work, it will distribute resources and bring about economies.

c. Planning

Nowhere is the Reagan approach more evident than in health planning. After more than a decade of federal support for planning (e.g., through President Johnson's "Regional Medical Program") and a "certificate of need" approach (e.g., through the Comprehensive Health Planning Act), the Administration has called for the abolition of all federal support and incentives for community and state health planning activity.

d. Regulation

The commitment of federal funds to long-term care, particularly through Medicaid (Title XIX) and to a lesser extent through Medicare (Title XVIII), coupled with scandals in the nursing home field, brought extensive federal regulatory activity particularly through the vehicle of the state Medicaid plan.

As part of a "pro-competition," "free enterprise" approach, new federal regulatory activity has come to a screeching halt, with current regulations under review.

Concomitant with efforts made to "cap" Medicaid is the move to relax those regulations which seem to generate costs. This philosophy is also evident in the block grant approach as well as in offers of a relaxed approach to state requests for waivers.

3. State Policy

States find themselves in an awkward situation. Having grown restive in a largely reactive role, they are being given the opportunity to exercise initiative since federal assistance will be less categorical, with fewer strings and more flexibility. There is but one problem; there will be fewer funding dollars though the needs are growing.

a. Resource Allocation

Traditionally in New York State, federal funds allocated through categorical programs were handled outside the normal budget process. These funds were perceived to be within the administrative responsibility of the executive branch of government.

The legislature, long suffering under such an arrangement, successfully received a Court of Appeals decision that federal funds should be subject to the normal legislative and budget processes. The victory has been pyrrhic, however, in that the legislature must bear the responsibility to meet even greater needs with relatively fewer federal dollars. The new flexibility is substantially less than might appear in the face of deeply entrenched institutionalized patterns of meeting human need, making themselves felt through strong trade organizations plus state offices which often attended their birth or at least nurtured them.

b. Locus of Decision Making

It is unlikely that New York State will do away with its franchising system in health. It came into being in the mid-sixties as a precursor to federal policy. There seems to be little support in this state for the Reagan pro-competition approach, at least in health.

Similarly, there seems to be substantial commitment to some sort of community system in long-term care. There are various experiments discussed in this volume under way (e.g., Robert Wood Johnson program in Buffalo, Monroe County Long Term Program, and the Rensselaer Channeling program) even as an interdepartmental task force is developing a statewide plan.

The structure, scope, policies, procedures, and values of such an approach have yet to be worked out. Among the critical issues to be addressed is the freedom of choice of the individual, the points of entry into the system, whether it will include private pay patients and whether or not it will merely be a gatekeeping system or one that generates services for the person in need.

Also at stake is whether it will be a local or state-administered program. This issue is closely intertwined with the proposed state take over of the Medicaid system.

4. Local and State Administration Issues

Local and state government issues are like two sides of a coin. They constitute reciprocal functions. The following are questions about administration which have no answers as yet:

a. System and Its Function

If there is to be a local system, where will authority and responsibility lie? What functions will be performed and by whom? Will participation be obligatory or the choice of the individual? Will it reach the private pay person? Will local dollars be used to support some or all of it? What will the relationship be of the private to the public sector, of ambulatory care to inpatient care, of social services to health services?

b. Planning and Administration

Will a local agency have responsibility to develop the system? Will it be an existing agency? Which one? What authority will it have? Will all "cases" be controlled by a single agency?

5. Non-Governmental

a. Sponsorship

Will there be room in the new long-term care system for many different types of sponsorship? What autonomy would remain with individual agencies? Would they have any control over their destiny? Would they be able to serve persons on the basis of decisions made in an institution or agency? What kinds of sanctions will they have to contend with?

b. Private Investment

Will the system depend on investment of private capital? Will all types of service be provided by proprietary interests? What financial incentive will be given to encourage such investments? What types of instrumentalities for quality control will be used?

c. Private Philanthropy

Will the system depend on private philanthropy? United Ways generally leave aging and long-term care activities to the government. Will their policy change and if so, why? Will agencies be able to serve persons within a cultural, social, or religious milieu? Will they be able to give preference to those constituents that sponsor them?

d. Trade Organizations

Trade organizations tend to reflect the needs and concerns of chief executive offices. They are a formidable force in the public policy arena. They also exercise leadership with their constituents. Will the trade organizations which represent the various aspects of the long-term care field be a force which is positive or negative? Will they foster cooperation or higher competitiveness?

6. Societal Values

President Reagan gives voice to an ethic quite different than that in which public policy has been rooted for the past 45 years. He promises to get government off our back. Since the New Deal, policy has been predicated upon the premise of a positive role of government fostering the well-being of people.

During this period there has been a constant movement to assure rights and to create entitlements for "at-risk people." The administration questions the very concept of entitlement and down plays, as paternalistic, the role of government in protecting people and their rights.

A number of specific value questions have risen to the surface in long-term care areas as in other areas; these are listed below.

a. Personal Responsibility

How much responsibility can and should an individual assume for his/her well-being? At what point should government intervene to assist people to meet problems, to provide for the future, to assure a safe investment, and to protect against harmful products?

b. Family Roles

In a time of four- and five-generation families, what is the role of the family in regard to its frail member? Who has responsibility to whom? Should family members bear great fiscal responsibility for the member when chronically ill and if so, who? And for which relative?

c. Social Insurance

Since the adverse selection phenomenon tends to preclude private insurance from entering the long-term care market especially in the instance of older persons, should the federal government extend the social insurance approach to it as it has to income and health care services through Social Security and Medicaid?

d. Welfare

At what juncture should government's welfare role be exercised in long-term care? What portion of a spouse's resources should be used to support his/her disabled partner?

e. Quality of Life

What is the quality of life to which disabled persons have a right? What quality control measures should we utilize? Should we have a federal, state, and local standard of quality?

Epilogue

The number of the chronically ill and disabled will grow. The long-term care field is relatively new and poorly organized. It is essential that those in it play a leadership role as society examines its values and government rethinks its responsibility. The most vulnerable of our society have little ability to speak for themselves.

REFERENCES

1. *The Need for Long Term Care.* A Chartbook of the Federal Council on the Aging. DHHS Publication No. (OHDA) 81-20704.

2. Fries, J. F. "Aging, Natural Death and the Comparison of Morbidity." *New England Journal of Medicine*, July 1980, *303*(3), 130-135.

3. *The Need for Long Term Care.* A Chartbook of the Federal Council on the Aging. Op. Cit. page 58.

Long-Term Care Systems Development in New York State, Part I

Robert F. O'Connell

Background for New York State's Long-Term Care Plan

Many have questioned why New York State was interested in developing a long-term care system plan as well as a channeling site demonstration project. New York was selected as one of twelve states to participate in the combined site and LTC system plan development process. Another 15 states have only a LTC system plan development grant. Some of those states are relatively new at planning initiatives, whereas New York State does, in fact, have a State Health Plan with a long-term care component and has had one for a couple of years. So the question is why should New York invest more time and energy in this area?

The rationale behind the State's decision to pursue the grant was its emphasis on the systems approach for this particular planning initiative. For the first time, policy level decision makers of all major state agencies would come together once a month to focus solely on long-term care system issues and attempt to reach decisions on LTC resource allocations for the next five to ten years. Though the need is expanding, the fiscal climate precludes significant expansion. In such a stressful time and faced with such hard decisions, the system development process is believed to be the process to bring the State closer to resolution. Obviously, it may not resolve every problem, but it may move the State one level closer to where it should be over the next few years.

New York State's immediate agenda in system development was stimulated by the National Long Term Care Demonstration project

---

Robert F. O'Connell is Deputy Director, Program Development and Evaluation, New York State Office for the Aging, Albany, N.Y.

which is funded and co-sponsored by the Health Care Financing Administration and the Administration on Aging. As was noted above, there is a dual focus to this project: essentially one focus is the operation of a local channeling site demonstration as part of an intensive research project; the second focus is the Long Term Care System Development project. In responding to the initial RFP, New York State responded to both the site and system development together and then subsequently also submitted a separate system development application.

The Need for a Systems Approach in New York State

Application was a cooperative venture of a number of State agencies under the leadership of the Health Planning Commission and the State Office for the Aging. Setting a framework for the current initiative necessitates going back over the past five years in which a number of efforts to improve and rationalize the ways in which the frail and elderly gain access to appropriate long-term care services were undertaken in New York State. Several long-term home health care programs were designed to extend the availability of comprehensive home care to clients who would otherwise require care within an institutional setting. The Monroe County Long Term Care project is testing the feasibility of providing a comprehensive assessment and placement service for all types of long-term care services through a non-profit agency structure. The State Community Services for the Elderly Program, administered by the State Office for the Aging, is providing supplemental state funds to target services for the frail and at risk elderly. The Coordinated Care Management Corporation program for the health impaired elderly of Erie County was funded by the Robert Wood Johnson Foundation. In New York City, the Department for the Aging has received funding through Medicare waivers to test a community-based delivery structure to provide a wide spectrum of both medical and social services. The New York State Long Term Home Health Care Program (nursing home without walls) has been operating for a couple of years. All of these programs represent a significant contribution toward improving the delivery of long-term care services to the State's frail elderly and other chronically disabled residents.

However, in spite of the considerable success that these projects have enjoyed, they suffer from one common underlying weakness, i.e., they have for the most part been undertaken not as elements of a comprehensive strategy to develop and manage long-term care resources but as discrete, individual agency responses to specific needs and problems. Unfortunately, the lessons that we have learned from them have not yet really led to a reshaping of the system in New York State.

During the next two decades, New York State will face a growing crisis in the area of long-term care. Multiple causes of this crisis are rooted in shifting demographic patterns, particularly in the growth of the older age cohort, 75 years and older. That age cohort will increase by 29% during the next 20 years, compared to a 10% increase for those over the age of 65. By the year 2000, one in 20 residents of New York State will be over the age of 75 years. If the present utilization pattern continues in terms of institutional resources, it will necessitate an increase of some 12,000 long-term care beds. As is true nationally, New York State's high expenditure levels preclude the expansion of the long-term care system in its current form.

More than any other population group, the nation's elderly need and use medical care. Per capita personal health expenditures for those 65 and over were $1,745.00, compared to $651.00 for those between the ages of 19 and 60, and $250.00 for those under the age of 19. Persons 65 years of age and over account for almost three times as many patient care days in general hospitals as do younger patients. Under the existing system in New York State, with its medical model and institutional orientation, total costs of serving the at-risk population are projected in 1984 to reach 2.6 billion dollars, about 49% above the current level. Nationally, in 1973, total skilled nursing facility costs were around $7.3 billion; in 1979 they had risen to $17.9 billion and they are projected by the end of this decade to reach approximately $76 billion if, indeed, the current system does not change. Obviously, government has reached the limit of its ability to pay long-term care costs at a time when the number of those in need continues to grow. Thus is created the urgency to explore the alternative long-term care systems.

As described in New York State's 1979 State Health Plan, three major problems pervade the long-term care system. These include: (1) insufficient services in a system lacking balance between institutional and non-institutional sectors and between the health and non-health services; (2) uncoordinated and poorly understood financial structures; and (3) inappropriate use of the services that do exist. A few specifics here: although the State as a whole has a large variety of community-based resources, there are many rural areas that have few if any. Even in New York City, there probably are some communities that would fall in the service-poor category. Procedures for entry into the long-term care system are not established at all. With the exception of Monroe County, there are no communitywide mechanisms to direct at-risk individuals through the maze of levels and settings. There is a multitude of payers (funding sources) for the long-term cadre of services, each with different eligibility criteria which confuse consumers and providers alike. Comprehensive uniform assessment tools applicable to all long-term care settings and services do not exist. State and federal policies continue to encourage the institutional side of the service patterns.

Nowhere in the United States have long-term care issues been under greater scrutiny than in New York State. During the past decade the State government has made unparalleled commitments of financial, administrative, and programmatic resources to address the growing problems of long-term care. In addition to the programs mentioned above, the State program of enriched housing is another one that comes to mind as one of the major initiatives. However, despite these efforts, long-term care has been characterized as a non-system in New York State. Entry into the system is haphazard with the client or family confronted by the bewildering array of agencies, programs, and eligibility criteria. Non-institutional health and social support services, although increasingly available throughout the State, are poorly understood and frequently underutilized.

It was in this context that New York State identified the Long Term Care System Development Project as a unique opportunity to reassess and begin to reorganize its entire long-term care delivery system, and to further develop mechanisms for improving and coordinating services across that system. Essentially the channeling resources have provided New York State with funding for one year. Technically the year commenced in October of 1980 and should have terminated in October of 1981. However, New York State received a technical extension to the end of the calendar year, and the activities described below and further expanded on in the next chapter occurred throughout the calendar year 1981.

The Structure of the Long Term Care System Development Project

The Long Term Care System Development Project consists of a number of components illustrated in Figure 1. These components are critical in the development of a long-term care system plan. The

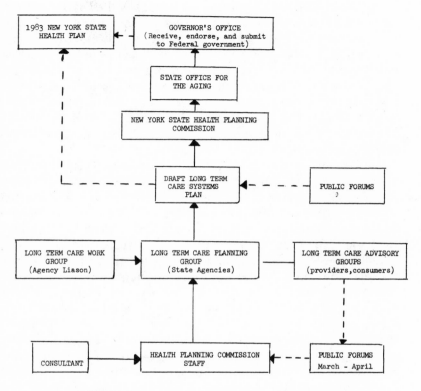

FIGURE 1. Long Term Care Systems Development Project

New York State Office for the Aging was the channeling grantee for the State; thus, it administers and has responsibility for both the local site demonstration in Rensselaer County and for the system development component at the state level. In terms of the system development component, the State Health Planning Commission has functioned as the lead agency and provides staff support to the Planning and the Advisory Groups. The major resource that has served as the decision-making body is the Long Term Care Planning Group which consists of the directors and/or deputy directors of the key State agencies. The directors of the State Office for the Aging and the Health Planning Commission co-chair the Long Term Care Planning Group. The other state agencies represented are: Department of Social Services, Office of Health Systems Management, Office of Mental Health, Office of Mental Retardation & Developmental Disabilities, the Department of State, and the Division of the Budget. These agencies have participated in monthly meetings with the commencement of bi-monthly meetings as we moved towards the final process. The group is responsible for developing a coherent policy framework, for setting specific program goals and objectives, for resolving policy issues that are common to several program areas, for restructuring individual parts of the delivery system, and for facilitating movement within the system as needs change. The major product of the Planning Group is a new State Long Term Care Plan.

In addition to the Planning Group there is a Long Term Care Advisory Group. The Advisory Group is comprised of other State agencies and various State councils such as the Home Care Council and, most importantly, various provider and consumer groups including the State Home Care Association, various unions, the Association of Homes for the Aged, the Area Agencies Association, the Statewide Senior Community Action Council, and others. The Advisory Committee has been convened from the beginning and has been involved in commenting in an advisory capacity on the products that have been generated. The structure has been very responsive to the needs and the desires of the Advisory Group. It is interesting how at the beginning of the process the Planning Group fell on one side of a position/option and the Advisory Group on the other. However, in many subsequent actions, the groups moved towards the middle in terms of the decisions that were made.

In addition, there is a Long Term Care Work Group which consists of the staff support from the participant agencies to the deputies or the directors that are represented on the Planning Group. This group does a lot of the hard and fast thinking, a lot of the staff work and preparation for the actual meetings of the Planning Group.

One of the components included in the process is a series of public hearings, one of which was planned early in the process to get feedback on what the concerns are and a second planned to lay out the basic directions of the plan. The first public hearing was held in New York City in April 1981, and a second public forum was held again in New York City later in 1981. The final Long Term Care System Development Plan will go through the regular Health Planning Commission process and be incorporated in the State Health Plan which is due again in 1983. It will also be reviewed by the Governor. Figure 2 represents the structure of the system plan development process.

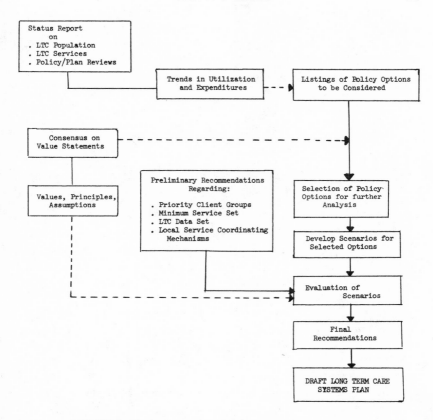

FIGURE 2. The long term care system plan development process

Long-Term Care Systems Development in New York State, Part II

Marilyn Pickett-Desmond

In the previous article, Mr. O'Connell outlined the general background for the Systems Development Project and a bit of the process. This article will provide some additional details on the process, particularly describing the kinds of policy options which have been under discussion. In addition, some early conclusions from the planning process will be presented.

The process involved initial consideration of fifteen policy options, a shopping list, so to speak, of strategies that might be considered. The Planning Group and the Advisory Group together chose nine of those for further consideration. The following section describes these nine selected options in order to provide an overview of what kind of issues are being considered. Since the process is still underway, the details on the recommendations to emerge from these discussions are uncertain, but some of the questions that have been raised in considering these options, and some of the initial determinations that have been made are, undoubtedly, informative.

What are the policy options considered? First is *A Prepaid Capitation Program for Long-Term Care*, which is known as the Social/Health Maintenance Organization, or S/HMO. This is a similar approach to the HMO, but it incorporates long-term care services in a prepaid capitation system. A demonstration program was initiated in New York City at the Metropolitan Jewish Geriatric Center, which is one of the first examples of this kind of approach in the country. The Planning and Advisory Groups are looking into the potential for this kind of an approach to determine whether we should pursue other demonstration programs within the state.

The second option is a difficult one: *Selective Reduction of Staff-*

. Marilyn Pickett-Desmond is Associate Health Planner, New York State Health Planning Commission, Albany, N.Y.

ing Standards for Institutional Care. New York State has standards for the levels of professional and paraprofessional health personnel staffing within long-term care institutions which exceed the minimum standards set by the federal government. The question is: should we re-examine our state standards? The background for these discussions comes from the observation that our current standards may be dated, and perhaps inappropriate. The standards now in effect were not developed based on a carefully designed examination of the needs of clients, but rather on a somewhat arbitrary set of guidelines. So the questions are: should we invest the resources to review our present standards and determine what an appropriate level of nursing staff should be? Should a case mix type of approach be used? What about staffing standards in developmental centers and psychiatric hospitals? Should they also be reviewed and revised?

Option three: *More Effective Utilization Controls.* This option involves an improved system of utilization and review which includes an improved assessment system at entry point into the long-term care system, and also a refocusing of continuing utilization review on those individuals who have a rehabilitative potential. Instead of trying to apply continuing utilization review resources among all institutionalized individuals, the system would be revised to identify those individuals as they come into a facility who have the greatest potential for rehabilitation, and to assist them to return to a lower level of care if possible.

Option four: *Dual Age Focus* for long-term care service eligibility is a concept that involves subdividing the long-term care population by potential need into two age categories. We currently have an approach in which we say that anyone over 65 is eligible for a certain number of services in the public sector. This option does not consider the fact that it is the subgroup age 75+ who may have greater need of supportive services in order to avoid institutional placement. The approach with this option would be to refocus the system so that there would be a subset of services available through public funding for those from age 65 to 75, which would include case management functions. However, those 75 and older would be eligible for an increased number of services. Essentially this would move the system away from trying to give a little of all types of services to everyone 65+, and try to focus on those populations which are most in need of the services. Again this is a way to try to deal with a limited amount of resources.

Option five: *Expansion of Community-Based Care.* This option looks at the feasibility of expanding a series of community-based services such as adult day care and personal care services. Under discussion are the issues that surround these types of programs: what has been the experience to date with utilization of community-based services; which services should be increased; what kind of control measures should be included if these services were increased?

Option six: *Expansion of Congregate Housing.* Similarly, what are the issues that we need to look at before we recommend the expansion of congregate housing? Unfortunately this option has limited viability because of the lack of finances which would be required to expand this kind of a program.

Option seven: *The Integration of Public Financing for Long-Term Care Services.* This is essentially the Senator Packwood Title XXI approach applied at the state level. Are there ways which resources from distinct funding streams could be "pooled" to some extent so that there would be essentially a combined pot of service money? This type of approach may allow decisions on buying services for those most in need, instead of on financial eligibility. The concept of pooling funds and utilizing them based on need rather than on eligibility criteria is a very difficult one to implement. It is, however, being tested by other states that are attempting to combine funds from several sources, and administer the funds through a single agency at the community level. The local unit makes the determination as to target populations and service utilization.

Option eight involves *Reorganization of State Agencies to Achieve a Single State Agency for Long-Term Care.* This is an interesting option because this was not among the original list of policy options to be considered. The Advisory Group indicated that while the State seems to have a lot of ideas on how providers at the local level should change their operations, attention needs to be directed to how the State can improve its own administration of long-term care. The general concept with this option is to combine the administrative functions which are now subdivided among five or six state agencies into a single agency for long-term care. The advantage to this would be that when administrative functions for long-term care are combined under a single roof, you can more readily begin to make decisions about the relative need for resources: where you are going to make an expansion, where you are going to have to cut back. Currently with public funding coming from the federal government through several different state agencies, New York State is essentially reactive instead of managerial. Decisions are not made as to where we are going to put our emphasis, but rather federal funding guidelines and eligibility criteria form the basis for much of our long-term care policy.

Option nine: *Community Alternative Systems Agencies.* This is a new program (the acronym spells CASA), which is similar to the "channeling" approach and includes assessment/placement, case management, and follow-up services for new entrants into the long-term care system. This has become the primary focus of the entire system development project and has become the focal point for much of the discussions about changes in the long-term care system. I will discuss this concept more fully a little later as it is an important issue in the plan development activities.

These then are the nine policy options currently under consideration. Each of these approaches has been analyzed in some detail and a scenario has been developed for each which looks at what would happen to the long-term care system if we follow this approach over the next five to ten years. What would be the impact of these kinds of policies, and what are the issues that we have to concern ourselves with before we pursue them?

In looking at these somewhat diverse approaches, there are four common themes emerging in the plan development process. These themes are going to serve as the framework for the plan, and for the long-term care policies which emerge from the planning process. The themes are as follows: First, *the growing demand for long-term care services should be met to the extent possible by the selective expansion of non-institutional alternatives. Institutional facilities should be used only when less restrictive alternatives are not appropriate or feasible.* Second, *demand for institutional services can and should be reduced through more effective gatekeeping at the point of entry, and the use of community-based care.* We are not just saying we are going to expand services, but rather, we are making a decision to reduce the demand for institutional care through increased utilization of community-based care. We are working toward tilting the system. Third, *the long-term care system must recognize and supplement the informal support system in order to effectively contain expenditures and enhance quality of care.* The issue has arisen repeatedly concerning the need to support, not supplant, the informal system that currently provides the majority of long-term support. Finally, *systems mechanisms must be developed to more effectively identify populations in need and to target services to those populations on a priority basis.* Long-term care services have not been targeted to those persons in greatest need in the past. Again we have been reactive. We place people in funding categories. We don't make decisions about priorities. We don't make decisions about target populations for particular services. We don't define who is appropriate for services.

These then are the themes emerging from the planning process. These four issues are a preview of the emphasis which will be developed in the recommendations. At this point in the process, the Planning and Advisory Groups have reacted to most of the option scenarios, and are beginning to develop specific recommendations.

As was noted above, the primary mechanism by which these themes are going to be operationalized is the Community Alternative System Agency, or CASA: the use of community-based co-ordinative services and a gatekeeping mechanism for the State's long-term care system as a means to make appropriate decisions on locus of care and types of services. An important aspect of the CASA approach is to consider more carefully what is the appropriate *site* of delivery for an individual moving through the system, and to consider options other than institutions. Inherent in the design of the program is to optimize the use of alternatives to institutional care when appropriate.

The discussions are focusing on establishing a statewide system of these CASA programs in each county or community. In developing this approach, there is movement towards a change in the relationship between the state and localities, just as the relationship between the federal and state governments has been changing within the past few years. What's being proposed is a more synergistic relationship between the state and local government, with the State encouraging localities to use innovation in developing these types of programs. The State can provide guidance and systems-kinds-of-management functions, but it is the local providers and governmental units which are familiar with the array of community services, understand the problems in those communities, and can develop approaches on how to overcome them. They can be the source of innovation in a program such as this.

What would be the specific functions of a CASA agency? Included are the (a) gatekeeping authority, or making determinations at the entry point to the long-term care system as to who is appropriate for institutional care, (b) identifying those individuals who could be more appropriately served in community-based care, and (c) assisting those individuals to utilize community services through case management procedures. An improved assessment system would be one of the basic requirements of these activities. Currently we do not have the tools needed to make these determinations, except in some of our demonstration programs. We do not have a statewide assessment tool that can help make the decision on appropriate *locus* of care.

Resource management may be an additional function of the community agency. CASA programs could participate in setting financial targets for total long-term care expenditures in the community, and essentially share in the financial risk for these long-term care service costs. The risk involved is an uncontrolled expansion of community-based care, beyond the capacity of the system. As you may be aware, some channeling-type of demonstration programs in other states which did not include some measure of control of total system costs have resulted in a very great expansion of community-based services. There is indeed a large potential demand for these types of services. What is needed is the rational system to make decisions on who should receive services based on relative need. That can be done more effectively if there is some type of budget for total service expenditures, and the risk of running over that budget is shared by those making decisions on service utilization.

Conclusion

This then, is the focus of the systems development project and a preview of the findings. Many of these concepts are now new—the expansion of CASA-type programs has been referred to extensively in long-term care policy in New York State at least since 1977. This time, however, I sense that we are moving ahead with some commitment and some energy, and part of it has to do with the change in the federal environment.

There is a concept in the literature of stress management which refers to the fact that a little bit of stress is good for you. It keeps you up; it helps you think; it makes you smart; it's called "eustress." However, if the stress continues to build, you fall into a situation called "distress" in which you are unable to make decisions. Right now the State is in an eustress condition. With federal cutbacks and increasing demand for services, there is pressure on the system. Administrative adrenalin is running at this point. The availability of the

Long Term Care System Development Project may serve as a timely means to focus the efforts of state agencies and providers, and to move towards establishing a *system* of long-term care.

Part II

DESCRIPTIONS OF SELECTED COMMUNITY-BASED, COORDINATED DELIVERY SYSTEMS IN NEW YORK STATE

Introduction to Part II

This section is devoted to the historical background and program descriptions of several initiatives for coordinating long-term care services in the State of New York. It begins with one of the oldest and most systematically evaluated systems in New York State—the Monroe County Long Term Care Program or ACCESS Project— and ends with some of the more recent efforts at systems develop-ment including the channeling grant and the Social/Health Maintenance Organization (S/HMO). The ACCESS program is a component of the Monroe County Long Term Care Program (MCLTCP). It was originally funded in 1975 and was incorporated in 1977 as a not-for-profit organization. Originally federally funded by Section 1115 of the Social Security Act, it operated through a Memorandum of Understanding with the New York State Health Department. These arrangements, as well as enabling New York Legislation, gave MCLTCP the authority to approve nursing home placements and home care services on behalf of all Medicaid recipients in Monroe County. Section 1115 federal waivers were also obtained by ACCESS to permit payment for home care services which previously had not been part of the New York State Medicaid System. Research results reported seem to indicate that it is a cost-effective program. Three long-term care demonstration projects developed after ACCESS in conjunction with the Monroe County Long Term Care Program, which have not as yet been evaluated, are also described. While they were not included in the conference, these demonstrations seem highly relevant and are illustrative of the sorts of spin-off programs which may result once a highly advanced long-term care system like MCLTCP is in place.

A second system, a bit older than ACCESS, is the Jamaica Services Program for Older Adults (JSPOA). It was begun in Southeast Queens largely as a grass roots organization with no federal funds. Currently it has multiple sources of funding and support. It is the only program described that did not get its start as a government sponsored demonstration.

A third program, the Nursing Home Without Walls program, had a somewhat different start: this program started in the New York State legislature in 1976.

The fourth program, the New York City Home Care Project, had still another beginning: it was started by the New York City Department for the Aging in 1979 with federal funds from HCFA and AoA, as well as with Medicare waivers.

The fifth program, the Erie County Coordinated Care Management Corporation, received private funding. It was funded by the Robert Wood Johnson Foundation.

The sixth program described is the Rensselaer County Coordinated Services Program, one of the AoA-HCFA National Long Term Care Demonstration Projects or channeling grants which is managed by the New York State Department for the Aging and which was begun in 1981.

Finally, lest you think the array of possible sponsors has been exhausted (for you will note that no two programs described in this volume have the same sponsor, though several share similar co-sponsors), the last and newest program is the Metropolitan Jewish Geriatric Center's Social/Health Maintenance Organization. This program was begun by a voluntary home for the aged with federal funding in 1981.

Despite the different sources of program sponsorship and funding and the different dates of origin, the programs described have many similar themes and problems, such as organization/coordination, case management, costs, and evaluation/assessment which will be further addressed in Part III.

It should be noted that very little in the way of evaluation is available. But from an evaluator/researcher's point of view the presence of seven slightly different programs of community-based, coordinated service delivery systems is something of a dream.

Assuming each program is serving a similar clientele, it should be possible to collect comparative data on all seven programs to determine which if any are more effective and efficient, especially in terms of costs and client outcomes.

Since many of the demonstrations are mandated to conduct research, e.g., the Rensselaer Channeling Program and the Erie County Program, perhaps some comparative data will be available at the time a next conference is planned.

The ACCESS Process:
Assuring Quality in Long Term Care

Gerald M. Eggert, PhD
Belinda S. Brodows, MSHyg, MA

Inappropriate use of costly and scarce health care resources takes many forms. It can occur in the overuse of emergency department services by patients whose conditions are not emergencies; in the increasing use of acute care hospital beds for patients who are not acutely ill; and in the use of nursing home beds for patients who are capable of living at home or at a facility providing a lower level of care. In each of these situations, patients are receiving more expensive care than they need—that is, care that does not contribute positively to their clinical or emotional conditions and that prevents others who need such care from receiving it. The inappropriate utilization of both acute care and long term care resources and the concomitant problem of cost containment have been well documented in the literature.[1-5]

The Assessment for Community Care Services (ACCESS) program of the Monroe County Long Term Care Program, Inc. (MCLTCP), in upstate New York has been addressing the problem of inappropriate utilization of health care institutions and the subsequent negative impact on long term care patients. The program's methodology includes identification of people who need long term care; assessment of client needs; development of service plans to meet those needs; and ongoing case management and monitoring accompanied by readjustments of service plans when necessary.

The purpose of ACCESS is to demonstrate alternative approaches to delivering and financing long term care to the adult disabled and elderly populations in Monroe County. The program's management process has been designed to enable individuals who need long term

Gerald M. Eggert is Executive Director and Belinda S. Brodows is Director of Research, Monroe County Long Term Care Program, Inc.

This article appeared in the February 1982 issue of the *QRB/Quality Review Bulletin*. Reprinted by permission of the Publishers.

care to receive appropriate high quality services in either nursing homes or in their own homes; to ensure that the services or placements that have been arranged are appropriate to clients' initial and changing needs; and to maximize the number of needy individuals who will have access to appropriate quality services at the least expense to the Medicaid program.

Structure and Objectives of ACCESS

In response to the need for ''an organized home care program for long term care patients,'' which had been identified in a 1975 study by the Finger Lakes Health Systems Agency,[6] the MCLTCP was incorporated in 1977 as a not-for-profit organization. The program was originally funded by Section 1115 of the Social Security Act and operated with responsibilities established through a Memorandum of Understanding with the New York Health Department and through contracts with the New York State and Monroe County Departments of Social Service. These arrangements, as well as enabling New York legislation, gave MCLTCP the authority to approve nursing home placements and home care services on behalf of all Medicaid recipients in Monroe County.[7] This authority enables the MCLTCP, through the ACCESS mechanism, to arrange for assessments to ensure that Medicaid recipients receive appropriate long term care. Section 1115 federal waivers also were obtained by ACCESS to permit payment for home care services which previously had not been part of the New York State Medicaid system.

The reduction of inappropriate utilization has been carried out through the use of a ''gatekeeping'' mechanism, whereby only those clients who meet ACCESS standards are recommended for a long term care bed. This mechanism was shown to be effective by a previous project conducted in Monroe County,[8,9] which indicated that an evaluation of clients' needs could be conducted by professionals in the community who already worked with them. Moreover, if adequate documentation of their needs was provided by the evaluators, the decision to seek long term care placement or home care services could be made by professionals, by the client, and by family members based on information in those documents.

Because the purpose of ACCESS is to use both the authority and waivers to demonstrate alternative approaches to delivering and financing long term care to the adult disabled and elderly populations in Monroe County, the following eight objectives were specified:

- To encourage persons needing long term care to choose home care rather than institutionalization when appropriate;
- To provide coordination and continuity of case management for long term care clients;
- To improve long term care assessment and review procedures;
- To collect data about the needs, service utilization, and appropriateness of placement of persons requiring long term care to facilitate future planning and evaluation for clients;
- To minimize inappropriate utilization of long term care resources;
- To reduce the number of Monroe County residents who are in acute care hospital beds beyond medical necessity while they await placement in a long term care facility;
- To reduce Monroe County residents' occupancy of long term care institutions by appropriate use of noninstitutional alternatives; and
- To reduce increased Medicaid and Medicare expenditures for individuals needing long term care (including both expenditures for long term care and for alternate care days in acute care hospitals while inpatients wait for long term care arrangements).

The ACCESS Case Management Process

The program's objectives have been carried out through a five-step process consisting of casefinding, assessment, determination of level of care, service plan development, and monitoring and reassessment.

Casefinding. The ACCESS process is initiated by referrals from community sources, such as families, physicians, community health nurses and agencies, and from hospital discharge planning staff. Referrals are stimulated through the distribution of brochures and other public relations materials; through interactions between ACCESS staff and professionals in the community and in hospitals; and through an extensive consumer-oriented outreach program that was carried out largely under the auspices of a federal government Administration on Aging grant.

Assessment. Depending upon the site of the referral, clients must consent to either a community assessment or a hospital assessment. Both types of assessment contain the same information and are based on a document called the Preadmission Assessment Form (PAF). A four-page form, the PAF is used for recording objective data about the patient, such as demographic information, medical data, functional status indicators, family support information, and a description of the client's required therapies.

When the client is an inpatient, the assessment is conducted by the hospital's discharge planning and nursing staffs. In addition, the client's physician completes the one-page medical summary. ACCESS reimburses the hospital a flat fee of $35 for completing the PAF and obtaining the client's consent for the assessment.

When a client is referred from a nonhospital source, an ACCESS staff member arranges for the assessment to be performed. If the client is in a long term care facility, the PAF will be completed by a member of the facility's nursing staff. When the client is in a domiciliary care facility (supervised living quarters without medical services) or at home, a community health nurse employed by either the Monroe County Health Department or the Visiting Nurse Service will perform the nursing evaluation (including a psychosocial evaluation). The medical workup is performed by a physician who will be reimbursed upon completion of the document. The cost of an average assessment for a community-based client, including all services, is $56.

Other reimbursable assessment services include financial counseling (to help both Medicaid and non-Medicaid clients use what resources they have to provide for their own long term care needs), in-home architectural review, housing improvement services to identify and modify any physical impediments in clients' homes, and social work consultations.

Determination of level of care. The case management system, which is designed to maintain continual contact with clients by the ACCESS program, begins when an individual is identified as a potential long term care client and is referred to ACCESS. When an assessment is required for either an institutionalized patient or one who has been referred from the home or from a domiciliary care facility, the ACCESS case manager works with the appropriate nursing and medical personnel to complete the PAF; the case manager also arranges for a financial counselor, occupational therapist, or social worker to complete other components of the PAF as required.

After the assessment is complete, the ACCESS case manager certifies the level of care needed by the client according to the five levels of care determined by the ACCESS program (see Figure 1). The level of care indicates both the type of long term institutional care as well as the equivalent level of home care services that are appropriate for each patient.

Once the certification decision has been made, the case manager works with the evaluator and client to determine the best site for the client to receive care. The client's preference is a major factor in the decision. Thus, when elderly clients prefer to remain in their homes, the case manager arranges for the completion of necessary forms and subsequent provision of services in the clients' homes. For those clients who require assistance but who lack a support system at home, the case manager arranges for nursing home placement.

When a client is eligible for Medicaid, the ACCESS case manager can approve the payment of Medicaid funds for nursing home

LEVELS OF CARE

Level 1, Minimal or No Needs

No further explanation needed.

Level 2, Domiciliary Care

Care for patients who require general supervision by nonprofessional attendants. It also includes minimal to moderate assistance with activities of daily living (ADL).

Level 3, Health Related

Care for patients who require minimal to moderate nursing evaluation and supervision. It also includes minimal to moderate assistance with ADL.

Level 4, Intermediate-Skilled

Care for patients who require skilled nursing service but not on a daily basis. It includes moderate to complete assistance with ADL. There may or may not be therapeutic and rehabilitative services.

Level 5, Skilled Care

Care for patients who require treatment involving daily skilled nursing care and/or daily rehabilitative services. As a practical matter, these services can only be provided in a skilled nursing facility when acute hospital care is not required or indicated.

FIGURE 1. These five definitions of long term care form the basis of the ACCESS case manager's recommendation for the type of care required by a client.

placement or for home care services up to 75% of the equivalent long term care costs. When the cost of home care services falls within 75% to 110% of institutional care, the care plan can be approved by an on-site monitor from the Monroe County Department of Social Services. If the costs exceed 110%, the care plan must be approved by the Deputy Director of Medicaid in the Monroe County Department of Social Services.

When a client is not eligible for Medicaid payment, the case manager assists the family in obtaining privately financed services. The ACCESS financial counseling service helps non-Medicaid clients allocate their resources to achieve maximum benefit.

Service plan development. A service plan is completed for all clients for whom home care services are recommended. This plan is developed by a community health nurse and documented on an Alternate Care Plan (ACP) form. A fee of $25 is paid by ACCESS for completion of the ACP, which accompanies the client's first PAF. The ACP specifies the home care services recommended by the community health nurse, such as "friendly visitors" to provide companionship for elderly clients who live alone; "respite care" to provide institutional or noninstitutional care so that families can be temporarily relieved of their caretaking tasks; "social transportation services" to enable individuals to receive other services as specified in the care plan; "home maintenance and heavy chore servcies" to perform maintenance on the client's house; "housing assistance" in the form of a temporary monetary rent subsidy to enable needy individuals to live in an adequate environment; and "moving assistance" to help clients who must relocate or move into suitable housing. The ACCESS case manager often assists the community health nurse in developing a plan.

Monitoring and reassessment. After ACCESS clients are placed in a nursing home or are receiving home care, they are monitored continually to ensure that the care being provided is medically necessary. As the clients' needs change, the home care services or institutional placement can thus be adjusted.

The mechanism of the monitoring system differs according to the site of the client's care. In nursing homes, an admission review is completed within five days of a client's admission. The review form, called the ACCESS Initial Form (AIF), contains the same functional status information as the assessment PAF. All AIFs are reviewed by the ACCESS supervisor to determine the appropriateness of admission.

Continued stay reviews, which contain information identical to that on the AIF, are completed by utilization review staff at intervals of 30, 60, and 90 days, and every 90 days thereafter, and are forwarded to the ACCESS supervisor. The supervisor evaluates the review and certifies the medical necessity for the client's continued stay in the institution. Improvement or deterioration in a client's condition may affect his or her placement and level of care.

Clients who receive services at home are monitored in several ways. First, to ensure that ACCESS can identify and respond to a client's changing needs, continual communication is maintained among the case manager, the community health nurse, health care providers, and the client's family. Second, case managers telephone clients who are not receiving Medicaid-reimbursed services every four to six months to monitor and respond to their changing needs. Third, a system of formal recertification of need is maintained for Medicaid beneficiaries through an abbreviated PAF form, called the home review form.

The home review form and revised ACP are completed every 120 days by the community health nurse after a visit to a client's home and are reimbursed by Medicaid at a rate of $32. These documents form the basis for formal recertification of medical necessity and readjustment of the care plan by the case manager. Finally, case managers provide an additional quality check by visiting clients at home or in nursing homes as needed.

In addition to ensuring that clients receive appropriate and high quality care through the case management monitoring process, the ACCESS program uses two other quality assurance mechanisms. First, a case management systems review committee meets several times a year to review records and to evaluate the effectiveness of the case management functions. The committee's findings are then used to identify and correct any existing problems in the system.

Second, quality of care in the ACCESS program is monitored by the Monroe County long term care review team, which is supported by the Monroe County Department of Social Services, and which has two major responsibilities: to approve Medicaid payment for individuals whose care plans fall between 75% and 110% of the equivalent institutional rate; and to monitor the quality of services provided to ACCESS Medicaid clients. Nurses for the review team randomly visit clients to ensure that the ordered services are being provided properly. This additional monitoring supplements monitoring by the case managers.

Outcome

Utilization. The ACCESS process has facilitated the provision of appropriate long term care services to approximately 9,500 persons from December 1977 to May 1981. Assessments during 1981 have averaged 390 per month with 70% of the referrals being made from hospitals and 30% from nonhospital sources.

Since the beginning of the ACCESS program in 1977, case managers have determined that 46% of clients referred from nonhospital sources have needed skilled level care, and 89% of these have been able to remain in their homes. For those clients referred from acute care hospitals, 76% needed skilled level care, and 36% were able to return home.

These statistics indicate a trend: in 1978, 81% of home assessments resulted in home placement; in 1979, this number had increased to 91%, and in 1980, to 92%. A similar pattern can be seen with respect to hospital referrals. From 1978 to 1980, the percentage of clients assessed in hospitals at the skilled level and who returned home increased from 19% in 1978 to 38% in 1979, and, finally, to 41% in 1980. In addition to the increasing numbers of individuals who required intensive, skilled nursing level care but who were able to return home, the number of clients who have been assessed annually has greatly increased over the past three years. In 1978, 2,878 assessments were completed for ACCESS clients; in 1979, 3,573 assessments were completed; and in 1980, 4,224 assessments were made.

These patterns are important because an increasing number of referrals has meant that more individuals who have needed long term care have been assessed and monitored through the ACCESS system. For clients, participation in the ACCESS program has enabled them to receive appropriate quality care, and, for the community, ACCESS has helped to assure that long term care resources are used appropriately by clients who need them.

The increasing proportion of functionally disabled people who have been able to remain in their own homes also has been a positive outcome of the program. Through ACCESS, clients have been offered a choice of where they would like to receive care; many have preferred to return or remain home. In addition, the ACCESS program has enabled the Monroe County community to develop noninstitutional home care resources. These home care services have been much less costly than the expansion of existing hospital or nursing home resources.

Cost. Finally, the ACCESS program has decreased the growth of Medicaid expenditures for recipients who need long term care. By substituting home care services for hospital or nursing home care, ACCESS has been serving more clients at a lower overall cost (see Table 1).

Since the initiation of the program, the number of Medicaid recipients has increased by 9%, total expenditures have increased by 30%, and the cost per recipient has increased by 20%. These figures compare to six similar comparison counties in New York State in which the number of Medicaid recipients has increased by only 1%; the average total expenditures have increased by 42%, and the cost per recipient has increased by 41%. Thus, although the number of Medicaid recipients served through ACCESS has increased more than in the other counties, both total expenditures and Medicaid cost per client have not shown similar increases.

The high growth rate of home health care in Monroe County (131% since 1978) in comparison with the other areas (57.2%) appears to be the reason for the lower rate of expenditure growth (compare data from Table 1 and Table 2). At the same time, nursing home expenditures have risen 5.7% in Monroe County compared with a fourfold increase of 23.1% in the comparison counties.

TABLE 1. Seven-County Comparison of Average Percentage of Change in Medicaid Costs and Beneficiaries for Clients $\geq$ 65 Years of Age from Pre-ACCESS Period (12/75-3/78) to Post-ACCESS Period (4/78-4/80)

County	Beneficiaries	Total Expenditures	Cost Per Beneficiary
Erie	− 10%	+43%	+59%
Broome	− 2	+35	+37
Onondaga	+ 3	+49	+44
Suffolk	+ 4	+47	+41
Albany	+ 6	+34	+26
Westchester	+10	+40	+28
Average (above)	+ 1%	+42%	+41%
Monroe	+ 9%	+30%	+20%

Reprinted from MACRO Systems, Inc. *Third-Year Evaluation of the Monroe County Long Term Care Program, Inc. 1980.* Reprinted with permission.

TABLE 2. Comparison of Percentage of Change in Medicaid Expenditures from Pre-ACCESS Period (12/75-3/78) to Post-ACCESS Period (4/78-4/80)

	Monroe County	Six Comparison Counties
Inpatient hospitals	+ 36.5%	+37.0%
Nursing homes	+ 5.7	+23.1
Health-related facilities	+ 22.3	+48.2
Home health care	+131.0	+57.2
Total	+ 18.9%	+32.7%

Reprinted from MACRO Systems, Inc. *Third-Year Evaluation of the Monroe County Long Term Care Program, Inc. 1980.* Reprinted with permission.

Because the average daily home care plan costs $25, the average daily nursing home rate is $50, and the average acute care hospital day costs $250, ten days of home care can be provided at the same cost as five days of nursing home care or one day of acute care. By increasing the number of clients who receive home care and simultaneously reducing the number receiving nursing home care, the ACCESS program has reduced the cost of long term care throughout the Monroe County Medicaid system.

Although the cost of services provided through the ACCESS program has not resulted in excessive increases in Medicaid expenditures, the costs of carrying out the quality assurance functions associated with case management also must be considered (see Table 3). The average daily cost of case management for all clients is $.95 per day. This cost varies according to both the referral source and client disposition. For example, case management costs vary from $1.13 per day, when the client is referred from the community, remains at home, and needs to have a service plan developed, to $.65 per day when the client is referred from the hospital and is admitted to a long-term care institution.

Development of a data base. In addition to ACCESS cost and utilization impact on Monroe County, the program also has been responsible for collecting substantial data on individuals who have received long term care. These data have been used to identify communitywide problems, such as the unequal admission rates to nursing homes of Medicaid and non-Medicaid clients; ACCESS data have revealed that non-Medicaid clients with family resources at home have been admitted to nursing homes.

Despite positive outcomes, however, a major problem remains. While ACCESS case managers must approve the level of care required by individuals seeking admission to a skilled nursing facility, ACCESS cannot decide who actually is admitted to an institution. The decision to admit remains with the nursing home which often accepts individuals from the community with lower disability levels (and with private financial resources) than those of hospitalized patients on Medicaid.

However, in the future, plans will be directed toward enhancing ACCESS's positive outcomes. The MCLTCP has recently received a Medicare 222 award which will enable ACCESS to waive the three-day hospital stay presently required by Medicare before it will reimburse patients for home care and nursing home care. The program also will be able to provide up to 100 days of additional skilled nursing benefits to individuals in their own homes and expand the interpretation of medical eligibility for nursing home benefits under Medicare. These new benefits will permit all ACCESS clients to receive reimbursement for additional long term care services.

TABLE 3. ACCESS Case Management Costs per Client in 1980

	Referred From Community	Referred From Hospital	Average*
Referred for home care	$411/year $1.13/day	$394/year $1.08/day	$405/year $1.10/day
Referred to a nursing home	$254/year $ .70/day	$238/year $ .65/day	$239/year $ .65/day
Average*	$398/year $1.09/day	$303/year $ .83/day	$346/year $ .95/day

*Based on weighted averages and therefore will not compute exactly.

Reprinted from MACRO Systems, Inc. *Third-Year Evaluation of the Monroe County Long Term Care Program, Inc. 1980.* Reprinted with permission.

REFERENCES

1. Entering a nursing home: Costly implications for Medicaid and the elderly. *Comptroller General's Report to the Congress of the United States.* General Accounting Office, Nov 26, 1979.

2. Krill G: Overstay among hospital patients. *Health Soc Work* 2(1): Feb 1977.

3. Manber MM: Patients with no place to go. *Medical World News,* Apr 14, 1980.

4. O'Shaughnessy C, Reiss K: *Long Term Care: Community-Based Alternatives to Institutionalization.* The Library of Congress Congressional Research Service, no. 1B 81013, Oct 1, 1981.

5. Sullivan R: Study says nursing home bed gap causes Medicare waste on elderly. *New York Times* Jun 11, 1979.

6. Finger Lakes Health Systems Agency: *Bed Survey Study.* Rochester, NY, 1975.

7. Laws of New York State 1977. Chapter 758: An Act to Amend the Social Services Law in Relation to Authorizing Social Services Districts to Conduct Residential and Medical Care Placement Demonstrations.

8. Williams TF, Hill JG, Fairbank ME: Appropriate placement of the chronically ill and aged. *JAMA* 226: 1332-1335, 1973.

9. Williams TF, Hill JG, Fairbank ME, et al: Evaluation-Placement of the Chronically Ill and Aged (unpublished project summary). Rochester, NY, Feb 1977.

Long-Term Care Demonstration Projects in the Rochester Area

James Fatula

The following are summaries of three projects dealing with hospital back-up of patients awaiting placement for long-term care services. These projects are important innovations in long-term care which are local initiatives but have a much broader potential. They were developed in collaboration with the Monroe County Long Term Care Program, Inc., described in the previous article.

1. The Long Term Care Capitation Project

The back-up problem—hospital patients who no longer need acute care and are awaiting placement for long-term care services—is a national problem. A background report prepared for the Department of Health and Human Services in 1981 estimated that Medicare and Medicaid pay for between one million and nine million hospital back-up days annually for patients who do not need acute care.

The problem is particularly acute in New York State which has the highest percentage of hospital beds occupied by alternate care patients in the country. The New York State Health Planning Commission estimated that in 1980 more than 7% of the hospital beds in the State were occupied by patients on alternate care status. In Monroe County, New York, almost 10% of the acute care beds are occupied by backed-up patients. Since Monroe County has one of the lowest ratios of acute care beds to population in the State, the back-up problem places enormous pressures on the effective functioning of the health care system in the county.

In response to the problem, the Rochester Area Hospitals' Corporation and the Monroe County Long Term Care Program, Inc.,

James Fatula is Director, Long Term Care Capitation Project, Rochester Area Hospitals Corporation, Rochester, N.Y.

developed a proposal through the New York State Department of Social Services to request section 1115 demonstration waivers from the Health Care Financing Administration.

The primary objective of this demonstration is to reduce the back-up of Medicaid patients in hospitals who would be more appropriately placed in a lower level of care. As a result, limited health care resources would be used more efficiently, and Medicaid costs would be reduced. The project proposes to introduce financial incentives and non-financial interventions to reduce hospital back-up. The financial interventions consist of two main portions: (1) the capitation payment system which will determine the payments to be made by Medicaid to the participating hospitals and (2) the case-mix system which will provide guidance to the hospitals as to the amount that it would be reasonable for them to pay as incentive payments to long-term care providers to encourage the prompt and appropriate post-hospital placement of enrolled patients. Non-financial interventions are characterized in two ways: (1) hospital-based efforts aimed at identifying elderly patients at risk of becoming backed-up and instituting measures to prevent or deter patients from becoming backed-up and (2) strengthening the working relationships among hospitals and long-term care providers in the care of the functionally disabled elderly.

Patients would be enrolled in the Long Term Care Capitation Project if they satisfy the following criteria:

a. Had an inpatient hospital stay in one of the participating hospitals.
b. Require SNF level care.
c. Had not received care in a SNF on an inpatient basis during the 90 days prior to the admission to the hospital which led to enrollment in the Long Term Care Capitation Project.
d. Medicaid will be a source of payment for long-term care services on discharge from the hospitals.

Patients who use only emergency room hospital services would not be enrolled.

Once enrolled, the patient would continue to be the responsibility of the hospital receiving the capitation payment for a period of one year from the date of enrollment, unless the patient dies or ceases to be eligible for Medicaid, in which case the capitation payment and the responsibility of the hospital would cease.

The hospital will receive a capitation payment from Medicaid for each patient enrolled in the demonstration. The capitation would start the day the patient went on alternate care status. The capitation payment would be set at some percentage (less than 100%) of the amount that Medicaid would have been likely to pay for the future care in the hospital of alternate care patients for some defined period of time.

The capitation payment would cover the hospital's costs for the alternate care stay to the extent that they exceed the average SNF per diem for the area. In addition, the hospital would contribute some percentage of the capitation payment to a contingency fund for special projects and for possible use as a reinsurance mechanism. Hospital interventions to prevent or deter patients from becoming backed-up would also be paid for from the capitation payment to the extent that additional expenditures are necessary. The balance of the capitation payment would be available for incentive payments to long-term care providers to encourage them to take the enrollees from the hospital as quickly as possible. The hospital would be allowed to retain any surplus resulting from the total of these payments being less than the capitation payment, and would be responsible for any excess payments over and above the amount of the capitation payment.

The capitation payment is not intended to cover the cost of acute care. The costs of acute medical care, either on an inpatient hospital basis, or on an outpatient basis, would be paid for as in the present system. If the patient is readmitted to a hospital and incurs an alternate care stay, those alternate care days would be paid for in the same way as the alternate care days in the original stay. If Medicaid is the responsible payor, Medicaid would pay the average SNF per diem for each day of alternate care stay, and the capitation payment would be used to cover a portion of any additional costs. If another payor is responsible for some or all of the days, then that payor would be billed as usual.

The long-term care providers would continue to receive their standard Medicaid payments from Medicaid directly. When they agree to accept one of the enrolled patients from one of the participating hospitals an agreement would be reached concerning the amount of incentive payment that the hospital would make to the provider for the care of the patient, and the length of time for which that payment would be made. The amount of the incentive payment would vary according to case-mix groupings.

When a patient is enrolled in the demonstration, Medicaid would pay the responsible hospital a capitation payment. The hospital would then have to decide how much of that capitation payment it is reasonable to expend to facilitate the placement of the patient. It would be possible to place some of the patients promptly with little or no payment from the pool of capitation money, but others may require substantial incentive payments to facilitate their placement and the total incentive payments for these patients may even exceed the total individual capitation payment. The expectation is that, on average, the cost to the hospital of the incentive payments would be less than the total amount of the capitation payments received less the amount needed to cover the costs of the unavoidable alternate care incurred by the patients and the costs involved in introducing interventions in the hospitals to prevent or deter back-up. Since the hospitals and long-term care providers have no experience in the determination of such incentive payments, some guidelines are needed to indicate how much would be reasonable for any particular patient. The case-mix groupings would provide this assistance. A patient would be assigned to a group based on a set of characteristics, and associated with that group would be a range of reasonable costs for that type of patient. The hospital would negotiate with the long-term care providers for the placement of the patient using the knowledge of which group the patient is in to assist with deciding the reasonable amount of the incentive payment, whether it should be paid for the entire year, and any other conditions that might be appropriate.

The ranges computed would be advisory to the hospital and would not constrain the flexibility to negotiate a higher or lower amount for the placement of any particular patient.

In addition to the financial interventions to encourage appropriate and cost-effective post-hospital placement of patients, the project would support a series of non-financial interventions in the hospital that would achieve this goal. The purpose of these efforts is to intervene early and aggressively at various decision points during the entire hospital experience of at-risk patients to control the inflow into avoidable alternate care stays. These interventions include: initiation of early discharge planning for at-risk patients; the use of interdisciplinary geriatric consultative teams (described below) to assist in improving the functional capacity of at-risk patients during the acute stay; more consistent referrals to other community programs, such as Strong Memorial Hospital's Long Term Care Program (described below); assessment, case management and referral services for at-risk patients who present in the emergency department; staging area for long-term care within the acute hospital; and psychogeriatric consultation services.

2. The Geriatric Consultative Team Project

A major recommendation of the Task Force on Long Term Care of Rochester Area Hospitals Corporation, in July 1981, to help address the serious and worsening problem of back-up of patients in acute hospital beds awaiting long-term care, was:

> to establish geriatric evaluation/consultation teams in each hospital which will provide assistance and recommendations for improving or maintaining the functional capabilities of patients at risk of back-up, and recommendations and assistance in the use of full range of long term care services in our community.

In response to this recommendation, staff members from seven hospitals and the Center on Aging prepared and submitted to RAHC a proposal for the "Geriatric Consultative Team Project," to undertake the above objective and to evaluate the effectiveness of this effort. In October 1981, the Project was approved for support.

Each participating hospital identified one or more staff members in each of the disciplines of internal medicine, nursing, and social work, to serve as its geriatric consultative team. These team members had had variable amounts of previous experience in care of the elderly and in dealing with long-term care. Monroe Community Hospital, in addition to having its own internal team, provided staff in the three disciplines to consult regularly with the teams of the other hospitals in an advisory and training function in geriatrics and long-term care. The Center on Aging of the University of Rochester provided coordination and clerical services and, through the Department of Preventive, Family and Rehabilitation Medicine, arranged to have careful evaluation conducted.

The Project limited its activities to patients admitted or in the Emergency Department aged 70 and older. This choice was made in order to focus on the group of elderly at highest risk of back-up, while accounting for an estimated 80% of all back-up patients. A short registration form was completed on each such patient. Each team screened the registration information and other sources of information as it might choose (Medical Record, interviews with staff) to determine whether the patient was at sufficient risk for ending up on alternate care awaiting long-term care to warrant a full geriatric team consultation. For each full team consultation, each team member reviewed the Medical Record, and as he/she deemed necessary discussed the patient with the staff members regularly involved in the care of the patient and/or saw the patient. A Consultation Form was developed and used for recording relevant information on the medical, nursing, and social characteristics of the patient, team recommendations, and follow-up information. Screening and initiation of full team consultations was accomplished within the first 48 to 72 hours after admission. In addition to the data provided from the registration forms and the full team consultation forms, described above, other sources of information used in the evaluation included RAHC weekly monitoring of the numbers of patients on alternate care status in all hospitals in Monroe County, a series of three intensive, countywide surveys of alternate care patients conducted at 10-week intervals, minutes of joint team rounds, and other documentation.

At the six hospitals which participated in this Project for the six months of January through June 1982, there was a total of 5,112 admissions of persons aged 70 or older, as reported on the Registration Forms. This represents 11% of all admissions to these six hospitals in the six-month period. From these 5,112 patients aged 70 or older admitted and screened for likely risk of ending up in a back-up status, a total of 372 were so identified and had full team consultations. These represent 7% of all admissions of older patients. The percent of consultations varied somewhat between hospitals, over the range of 2 to 11%.

The measures of outcomes that we have in this Project to date indicate that, associated with the period of concentrated team effort, there has been a steady, sustained decline in numbers of patients on alternate care in the acute hospital which is only partly explained by the opening up of additional skilled nursing beds. The overall prevalence of patients on alternate care has been reduced in six months from 13% to 9% of hospital beds. The evidence from analysis of the various data available in this Project points to a number of aspects and recommendations of the team activities which have most probably contributed to success in helping older patients on alternate care leave the acute hospital for home or less intensive care settings than skilled nursing. A series of obstacles or systems issues have been identified which, if effectively addressed, should help even further to make earlier and more appropriate discharges possible.

3. *The Long Term Care Demonstration Program at Strong Memorial Hospital*

The Long Term Care Demonstration Program at Strong Memorial Hospital of the University of Rochester was designed to address the health care needs of those aged individuals in hospitals awaiting nursing home placement. By re-focusing care that these hospitalized elderly are receiving, it is hoped that their level of care can be lowered and they can avoid skilled nursing home placement.

The target population includes those individuals who had been functioning independently in the community until a recent acute health problem resulted in hospitalization. Over time, the health problem had been stabilized; however, they did not adequately achieve their previous level of functioning.

The health focus of the Program is that of self-care. The Program emphasizes teaching clients new ways to be independent. This begins with an assessment of the current functional level, as well as a determination of the functional level necessary for discharge. Care addressing the needs and goals of each individual, as well as all the therapies, are performed on the unit and integrated into a daily schedule.

Staffing on this 20 bed unit consists of a multidisciplinary team which includes nursing, physical therapy, occupational therapy, social work, medicine, dietary, speech, and activities therapy. Nursing on the unit is unique in that there is a high percentage of professional nurses on staff. The professional nurse, as the primary nurse, coordinates the multidisciplinary approach and assures that the treatment and care programs, as delineated by all health care providers, is implemented in a consistent, comprehensive manner.

The client and his family or social support system are involved in developing a realistic discharge plan. While preparing for discharge, a special assessment is done which includes having the client go home for an afternoon with his or her nurse. Special attention is given to evaluating client capabilities on the stairs, in the kitchen, and in the bathroom. Any problems that arise are addressed on the unit, by the entire team, prior to actual discharge.

The Long Term Care Demonstration Program has additional goals beyond those of patient care. Numerous educational and research projects are underway by both nursing and medicine to help promote the concepts of gerontological health care. Professional development toward achieving high quality standards of practice for all health care providers caring for the elderly is also taking place.

The Program has been operational since July 1982, and holds much promise for decreasing the number of individuals awaiting nursing home placement. Thus far, through the concentrated efforts of the Program's team, elderly individuals have been able to avoid skilled nursing facility care and have returned either to home or to a lower level of institutionalized health care.

The Jamaica Service Program for Older Adults (JSPOA) and the Southeast Queens Consortium of Aging Services (SEQCOAS)

Alice Watson

The Jamaica Service Program for Older Adults (JSPOA) is a community-based voluntary agency offering supportive services to the approximately 74,000 elderly residents of Southeastern Queens. JSPOA has from its inception been concerned with the development of services that will help senior citizens to remain as active members of the community. The organization coalesced from an earlier community effort begun in 1970 by local organizations, agencies, and churches that investigated the need for more adequate, low-cost housing for the elderly and formed a coalition that sponsored the construction of Conlon-Lihfe Towers, a 216-unit facility built under private auspices as a turnkey operation and now managed by the New York City Housing Authority.

Once it became evident that the housing would come into being, the coalition began to struggle with a problem that has remained a central concern ever since—how to evolve a continuum of services to enable seniors to remain in the community? For while the community had succeeded in developing housing that would allow older persons to remain in their community, other essential services were unavailable. At that time, only two senior centers served the area. There were no geriatric health clinics, few recreational programs, no educational or transportation services for older people, few in-home services (other than for Medicaid eligibles), and no programs to promote safety, a primary concern of the elderly.

In 1972, the efforts of this coalition lead to the creation of JSPOA as a demonstration project sponsored by the Community Service Society of New York with funds from Title III of the Older Ameri-

Alice Watson is Executive Director, Jamaica Service Program for Older Adults, Queens, N.Y.

cans Act. At the heart of JSPOA were the seniors themselves as members of the Senior Citizens' Advisory Council; seniors were to help set priorities for the agencies serving Southeast Queens and assist in planning and implementing the new programs that were to develop during the 1970s. From the beginning, JSPOA emphasized an active partnership by caregivers and older persons with a motto, "A total community working together to serve its elderly."

One immediate result of this partnership was that the older persons pushed agencies hard to explore ways of developing services that were difficult to provide and fund. During the 1970s, new health care facilities were developed, homecare and home delivered meals expanded, and a joint transportation program among a consortium of agencies developed. The development of programs often required a mixture of tenacity and patience because of the long time between identification of need and funder response. For example, older persons participating in the initial JSPOA committees in 1972 identified safety as a major concern of seniors. Although JSPOA was able to develop a modest program through its resources and volunteers, it wasn't until 1978 that significant funder support was obtained for this service.

The good news for older persons in Southeast Queens was that programs expanded and seniors had a vital role in planning and implementing these services. The bad news was that economic conditions in the neighborhood became worse as did the problems of fragmentation and service limitation.

In a Brookings Institute publication, *Setting National Priorities: the 1979 Budget*, the authors maintain that new services and urban policies have improved the quality of life for the majority but

> they have imposed social and economic costs on the minority of people who live in areas of concentrated poverty. These people have more unemployment, more crime, more inadequate housing, lower-quality public schools and far less desirable neighborhoods than most urban Americans.

The agencies of Southeast Queens are acutely aware of the human costs associated with deteriorating local economic conditions. The problems of housing and poverty are particularly acute, and crime against the elderly has been a problem of increasingly large proportions for at least the last decade. Countless numbers of the aged are virtual prisoners in their own homes, self-confined victims, many having endured multiple incidents of violence against their person and property and fear going out into the streets.

As older persons in Southeast Queens faced serious worsening environmental conditions, our agencies experienced a new type of long-term community care challenge as participants and clients aged while our programs evolved. Our challenge became increasingly how to coordinate the multiple services—homecare, transportation, medical care—that were needed to support the determination of these older persons to remain in the community. Furthermore, an essential part of JSPOA's experience was the contribution that older persons made to service planning and delivery, to each other, and to their community. For the older old, the barriers to this participation became increasingly severe. For example, one agency in Southeast Queens struggled with the problems of an over 80 senior who had become blind but was determined to maintain her weekly participation in local planning board activities. This required arranging volunteer escort and transportation and while continued participation was vital to her and the committee's well-being, lack of funding for this within existing funding streams made the ongoing provision of this service extremely difficult and required creative and cooperative efforts.

By 1978 it had become more and more difficult for JSPOA's informal committees and task forces to arrange for coordination of services, especially for the frail, vulnerable, older persons requiring multiple services who were the growing concern of most of our agencies. Because of changes in the Administration on Aging funding priorities, it became increasingly difficult for JSPOA to obtain funds to maintain these activities.

An ongoing strength of JSPOA has been its ability to evolve organizational structures to effectively utilize the commitment of seniors and agencies to seek and to receive funding support when conditions require new approaches. In 1978 JSPOA received funding for an AoA Title IV-E Model Project as part of their long-term care program. The project, SEQCOAS, the Southeast Queens Consortium of Aging Services, had a goal of creating a more formal structure to plan and coordinate services to the vulnerable elderly. This structure was to be supported with electronic data processing capabilities.

A major organizational challenge for SEQCOAS was how to organize the commitment of agencies within a structure where participation was voluntary. When I am asked why agencies join SEQ-

COAS, my answer sounds simple—commitment to serving older people better, which is the power to be found at the community level. But in a voluntary consortium, this commitment is a perishable commodity that must be energized and reinforced by tangible successes. The power that we all recognize—the money and the mandate—is at other levels. The inability of a voluntary consortium to mandate is a continuing source of difficulty; it is also a potential for strength, for it forces the selection of realistic projects with clear benefits to member agencies that can be implemented by agencies using resources from within their own funding streams. A fact of life SEQCOAS confronted is that while each funding stream talks about coordination and service integration, there are very few national or individual funding stream mandates that support or reward organizational efforts to coordinate services with other funding streams. The formal mandate of the Older Americans Act and Title XX Program to give information, referral, and access services to older persons is the main exception. As dissimilar as a large hospital, a highly computerized social security agency, and a small nutrition site are, they confront almost exactly the same problems as they seek to refer vulnerable, frail, older persons to other agencies in the service delivery network. The attempt to address these common problems became the core around which our definitional, case management, and information collection activities would be built.

Since the division of labor among agencies in a voluntary consortium is crucial, for SEQCOAS the task was to develop a system of participation for 30 health, income maintenance, and social service agencies that differed in size, resources, mandates, and missions. This was accomplished by the negotiation of agreements concerning five options for participation in ways most appropriate to each agency. The five levels included two that are mandatory for all agencies and which focused on development of a common language, collection of baseline information, and establishment of the capability to document gaps in service. The three additional options involved using the SEQCOAS computer to support service provision and analysis.

The task of developing a common language with agencies from different funding streams was difficult and the complexity threatened at times to overwhelm the project. The assignment became more manageable when the committee decided to focus on the common elements in a long-term continuum of care for vulnerable older persons and to specify areas where a common language was essential for consortium activities; for example, a referral from a hos-

pital's social service department which required communication between this hospital and agencies providing home health, home
maker, escort, and transportation services. When we started the
process our goal was to get each agency to call an elephant an elephant and a squirrel a squirrel but soon we modified our goal to be
happy if we could get each agency to call an elephant a squirrel. We
succeeded in this more limited goal and developed a commonly
shared graphic of the referral process and network-approved common definitions for information, referral, advocacy, escort, transportation, and home care.

The definitional approaches of SEQCOAS through its committee
on Integrated Service Delivery took a great deal of effort and tenacity to develop. SEQCOAS had to struggle to come to grips with
language and communication. Figure 1 shows a graphic portrayal of
communication within funding streams.

SouthEast Queens
ConsortiumOfAgingServices

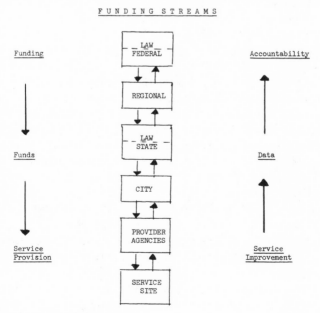

FIGURE 1. Funding streams

Figure 1 conveys how communication between service agencies and funding agencies is profoundly influenced by the geographic and bureaucratic distance between them. In general, regulations and language concerning program accountability flow down from funders, and data concerning service provision flow up from service providers to funders. These funding streams are "where each agency lives"; depending on the type of funding, each agency will have a different mandated service language.

At the various program levels—Federal, Regional, State, City, Service Site—there is very little horizontal communication between agencies in funding streams even when these streams offer the same service.

The designation "law" as noted in the Federal and State boxes in the chart emphasizes that agencies must, to receive funds and maintain accountability, follow the mandates that are communicated to them by laws and regulations. It points up universal awareness among members concerning the great impact of these rules and regulations upon agency planning and service delivery activities. These regulations specify:

—what services are offered, what they are called, and what measures will be used;
—how many clients can be served, and with what frequency;
—who is eligible for service.

Adding to the above, it is evident that even within funding streams there is often considerable confusion concerning service definitions. Often the funders, emphasizing accountability, have one interpretation while provider agencies, emphasizing service, have another. The development of this graphic has helped to identify some of the major complexities facing this multi-funded consortium.

Figure 2 deals with *network communication*. The essential nature of SEQCOAS network communication is horizontal communication among agencies in different service systems, but all committed to a common goal of improving services to older persons. In order for this communication to take place, it is necessary to develop a new common network language concerning target population, common service definitions, and unit measures.

SEQCOAS agencies have attempted to create a vehicle capable of promoting two-way communication between local and bureaucratic agencies. They are convinced that what has been accomplished at

SouthEast Queens ConsortiumOfAgingServices

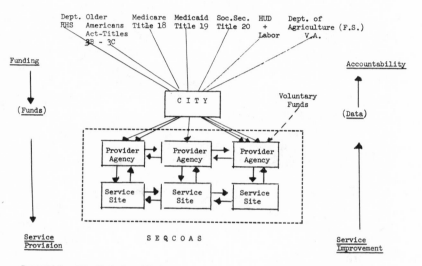

FIGURE 2. Network communication

the local level should be capable of being translated into changes in policy, funding priorities, rules and regulations, and administrative structures of higher level government agencies. Thus the lateral communication that has formed the basis of JSPOA's past success could be expanded to include improved vertical communication between funding agencies and service agencies and diagonal communication between local service agencies with information about specific clients and funders with resources in those needed areas.

The organizational and definitional activities of SEQCOAS allowed agencies to better communicate with each other. The shared concern was for the vulnerable clients who are unable to navigate the existing system because of individual agency mandates that allow response to only part of their problems, with no agency taking the responsibility for developing and implementing an effective care plan. These older persons often do not enter the system, drop out if they do, or may be unnecessarily institutionalized, when with coordinated services they could have remained in the community.

In an effort to move toward a service delivery system which would respond more effectively to these needs, SEQCOAS developed a project of interagency case management.

Unlike other case management systems in which the responsibility for case management is mandated by a government agency or other defined body, this project emphasized the *interagency* and *voluntary* nature of the system. No new staff were hired (with the exception of a Case Management Coordinator), nor were resources available for the case managers to purchase services, as is often the case in other systems. Each participating agency would designate a worker to be a case manager in the project. All member agencies were given an opportunity to participate, and SEQCOAS staff worked hard to ensure an appropriate mix of agencies to include: hospitals, social service agencies, mental health agencies, home care agencies, and senior centers.

Case managers take ultimate responsibility for assessing an individual client's needs, arrange for services, do follow-up as appropriate, and insure that the full needs of the individual are being met. All participating agencies agreed to use and help develop common forms for the collection and sharing of information either through direct access to a central computer or in team case planning and review meetings.

With everyone concerned about the issue of confidentiality, all affected parties, agencies, and representatives of the senior population developed a policy statement that ensured the dual goals of protection of client rights and the enhancement of service capabilities.

The case management system now in operation for a sample of our frail, vulnerable population has already been of value to case managers, to their clients, and to the consortium because we are beginning to collect information crucial to our ongoing service planning activities.

Information Systems to Support Case Management

The key element of SEQCOAS's information collection and distribution activities was evolving a realistic picture of the contributions that computers can make to service delivery, planning, and the costs associated with these benefits. Many in SEQCOAS were either in awe of the computer or suspicious; in any case, most expectations were unrealistic. A major turning point for the consortium was when members perceived that computers do not deliver services or make decisions. Our information collection capabilities improved significantly as we defined the role of the computer as assisting direct service providers to carry out their commitment to serve clients and to provide information to planners about frail, vulnerable, older persons that is not currently available.

With the assistance of case managers, SEQCOAS developed a client tracking system that is simple and less costly than other systems and that has several innovative features to support case management. For each vulnerable, at-risk client who enters the system, SEQCOAS' central computer selects data from the assessment and service planning forms to create and accumulate a one-page summary of planned client services. Information is presented concerning priority of service—emergency, high, normal—the agency or natural supports providing service, and which types of access services are required. Workers then update the final two categories on the service summary—current status and service outcome. As a result, simple one-page summaries concerning all clients' progress through the system are available at any given time.

We are pleased that the case managers now tell us that the information system does help them to plan and manage services to vulnerable, frail, older persons.

Policy Questions

A major contribution to the success of JSPOA has been that we have learned to listen and our staff and committees have always been willing to explore anything that might work and to build not only on what we have learned and accomplished, but also upon what has been learned from other service systems or geographic areas. A major problem we and other community projects confront is that while a wide range of sophisticated and innovative community long-term care approaches are currently being demonstrated, the field has lacked the ability to share information in ways that can lead to widespread replication of innovative ideas. Thus we reinvent the wheel not because of a desire to do our own thing—although that sometimes occurs—but because of historical and organizational barriers that often overwhelm the goal of utilizing the achievements of others. Some of these barriers include the facts that:

- It is far easier to obtain a large amount of money to implement a new project than to obtain a small amount of money to replicate an approach that another agency has already demonstrated.
- It is, at the community level, usually easier to obtain funding for a new demonstration project than to receive additional funding to expand and build upon the achievement of an existing project. The pattern of "three years and out" for community-based projects is an all too familiar pattern.
- Researchers and direct practitioners have historically operated in relative isolation from each other and as a result both groups have missed opportunities to achieve mutually supportive relationships.
- Much of the literature on long-term care demonstration appears written for *Science Digest* when what communities really need are articles from *Popular Mechanics*. We particularly need simple, concise descriptions of technological or organizational improvements that can be implemented by communities for relatively little money and an outline for step-by-step development of these new approaches.

Ironically, the movement to coordinate and integrate community long-term care services is itself becoming fragmented. The challenge we all face is to bring the various approaches together—government and foundation funded, mandated and voluntary, and direct service provision and service coordination—in a way that can transform parallel, isolated improvements into a cogent body of knowledge about effective long-term care approaches. I believe what we have learned at JSPOA can contribute to this process with Long-Term Care Centers taking a leading role.

I am glad to report that with all of our emphasis upon multiple problems, I can cite an evaluation project that has had multiple benefits. A short-term evaluation of JSPOA was carried out under contract with the Federal Council on Aging by JWK International Corporation.

At JSPOA we benefited from the opportunity to take time out from our daily management efforts to analyze in more detail where we have been and where we are going, and we received a final report that helped crystallize our accomplishments, problems, and policy issues that extend far beyond Southeast Queens. The Federal Council received the same analysis as part of a wider effort to study community-based aging service systems and will be able to study our experience with those of others within the same evaluation framework. The Columbia University Center for Geriatrics and Gerontology has completed a similar evaluation of SEQCOAS, and we look forward to obtaining similar benefits from their efforts.

There is a need in the community-based, long-term care movement for the same type of cooperative efforts that have channelized JSPOA and SEQCOAS and a similar need for both horizontal and vertical integration of efforts. JSPOA experiences on a weekly basis the need for horizontal integration among community projects across the country, for we receive requests for technical assistance that we cannot respond to and we require knowledge of other projects that we cannot obtain.

The need for vertical integration is reflected in this conference, and perhaps we can now take steps toward a more formal ongoing relationship between us to explore joint efforts to improve our programs and to identify and pursue policy issues that we share regardless of whether our source of funding is federal, state, agency, or local or comes from a private foundation.

There is a national concern about the growing cost of institutionalization and a population with an increasingly large proportion of older persons, especially the older old. Demonstration projects such as channeling are attempting to demonstrate that rationalization of the existing service system can help keep older persons in their communities and thereby lower institutional costs. We believe that community organizations such as JSPOA can and must make a contribution to service improvement projects of that type. Perhaps the greatest contribution is the observation that there is nothing magical about the concepts of coordination and service integration; improved, integrated services come about not because of the power of ideas but because of commitment of older persons to remain in their communities and of direct service providers to help them. Although it is almost inconceivable to think of improving services to those in need without encouraging innovations and policy input from direct service providers, this is what happened all too often in the 1970s. We talked too much about MIS, management by objectives, Program and Budgeting Systems and not nearly enough about communities, their needs, their strengths, and their natural support systems. A major asset of any community service organization is its continuing face-to-face contacts with older persons—both as clients and participants. Community agencies delivering long-term care services have a wealth of knowledge about their clients for they see them in their homes and in their neighborhoods. They realize the real need is not to reduce institutional care when it is needed, as it often is, but to provide integrated community services when they offer a viable alternative. JSPOA's success has been built upon its commitment to and involvement of older persons and the creation of a partnership of agencies with similar commitments.

Given the magnitude of the task being undertaken, we believe that all levels of government, foundations, and communities must work together so that what is known and has been accomplished at the local level can be translated into changes in policy, funding priorities, rules and regulations, and administrative structure at all government levels. If such a partnership is expanded, I believe that local initiatives being described at this conference can be expanded and enhanced and can contribute to the development of a cogent body of knowledge concerning what does and does not work to improve community-based, long-term care services.

Nursing Home
Without Walls Program

Bill Mossey

What It Is

The Nursing Home Without Walls Program provides nursing home level care to disabled, chronically ill, and invalid patients who are medically eligible for placement in a residential health care facility. Contrary to the usual practice of requiring a patient to conform to the programmatic mandates of providers of service, the Nursing Home Without Walls Program is tailored to the needs of each individual patient. Indeed, Nursing Home Without Walls' unique design can result in the savings of millions of health-care dollars, since it serves the same target population as institutions at about half the cost. At the same time, it allows for delivery of care in a home setting, where the patient is happier and more comfortable than in the institutional setting.

The Name

The Program was named Nursing Home Without Walls since nursing home level services are provided in a non-institutional setting. It is not necessary for a patient to be in a nursing home in order to receive nursing home level services; hence the name, Nursing Home Without Walls.

History

New York State Senate Health Committee Chairman Tarky Lombardi, Jr. developed the initial Nursing Home Without Walls legislation in 1976; over the next two years, the concept was refined and was ultimately signed into law as Chapter 895 of the Laws of 1977. It became effective April 1, 1978. Among the factors that led

Bill Mossey is Director, New York State Long Term Home Health Care Program, New York State Department of Social Services, Albany, N.Y.

Lombardi to seek this new approach to providing long-term health care were:

- Public health reimbursement mechanisms were geared toward the support of institutional care. This resulted in patients being prematurely institutionalized and often maintained in an institution long after it was necessary, although the patient would have preferred to be at home.
- The increased average life expectancy of individuals and the increasing percent of New York's population age 65 and older. For example, the average life expectancy has increased from 45.6 for males and 49.3 for females in 1900 to 69.9 for males and 76.9 for females in 1980, an increase of 53% and 56% respectively. The percent of the total population age 65 and over has increased from 4.8% in 1900 to 11.7% in 1980.
- The rapid rise in health care costs. National expenditures for nursing home care more than doubled between 1974 and 1978 according to the U.S. Government Accounting Office. In New York State, long-term institutional care consumes the largest percentage of public funds spent for health care. Medicaid pays for about 80% of the cost of long-term care in New York, while Medicare pays approximately 3%. Private and other sources accounted for 17% of these payments between 1977 and 1981.
- The occupancy rate for long-term institutional care in New York has exceeded 96% for several years. Thus it is often impossible to find a long-term care bed for a patient who could otherwise be discharged from an acute care facility.
- Recent studies by the federal government have found that 20 to 40% of the nursing home population were inappropriately placed and could well be cared for at less intensive levels of care.

Components of the Legislation

Patients

- The program must be offered to all Medicaid-eligible patients being considered for residential health care facility placement;
- Private pay patients are eligible for the program;
- Admission to the program is based on a comprehensive individual assessment of the patient's health, sociopsychological

status, and home environment. It is available to those patients who are medically eligible for a residential health care facility.

Budget

• Expenses for patients admitted to the program cannot be expected to exceed 75% of the local annual average Medicaid costs for maintaining the patient at a comparable level of care within an institution.

Providers

• Services to the patient are coordinated and managed by a single agency on a 24-hour, seven-day-a-week basis;
• Providers must offer comprehensive services comparable to those offered by residential health care facilities;
• Residential health care facilities, certified home health agencies, hospitals, and local health departments may apply to become providers.

Financial Savings

The Nursing Home Without Walls Program has proven that residential health care facility services can be provided to patients in their homes at a cost considerably less than that in an institution.

A. Comparison to Skilled Nursing Facilities

The Nursing Home Without Walls rate represents expenditures of less than 50% of the SNF rate—saving over a quarter of a million dollars for 270 patients in November 1980.

	Average Monthly Costs (November 1980)
Patients in a Skilled Nursing Facility	$ 1,955.72
Patients in Nursing Home Without Walls	968.12
Savings per Patient in Nursing Home Without Walls	$ 987.60
×	×
SNF level patients served in November 1980	270
=	=
Total Savings for 270 Patients	$266,651.00

B. Comparison to Health-Related Facilities

Nursing Home Without Walls patients are served at a cost of 69% of the cap and only 51% of the HRF rate, a savings of over $116,000 for 194 patients in November 1980.

	Average Monthly Costs (November 1980)
Patients in a Health Related Facility	$ 1,237.96
Patients in Nursing Home Without Walls	636.92
Savings per Patient in Nursing Home Without Walls	$ 601.04
×	×
HRF level Patients served in November 1980	194
=	=
Total Savings for 194 Patients	$116,601.00

C. Comparison to Acute Hospital Care

Many patients remain in hospital beds long after they actually require acute care because there are no available residential health care facility beds to which they can be discharged. The average cost for unnecessary hospital care in the counties which have Nursing Home Without Walls Programs was $16,953 per patient. The November 1980 Nursing Home Without Walls patients included 37.4% or 174 patients who were referred from hospitals. If they remained in an acute care facility for a similar period of time, the cost for this unnecessary care would have been (174 × $16,953) $2,949,822. The average Nursing Home Without Walls cost for the same period was (174 × $1,865) $324,510, a difference of $2,625,312. This shows that the cost savings can be dramatic when discharge planning is done early.

Patient Profiles

- Average Age of Nursing Home
  Without Walls Patients   73.8
  (Ages range from 2 to 107)

- *Patient Sex*

Female	76.3%
Male	23.7%

- *Source of Referral*

Hospitals	37.4%
Residential Health Care Facilities	1.9%
Community Agencies	52.5%
Family Members or Self	8.2%

- *Level of Care Upon Admission*

Skilled Nursing Level	61.6%
Health Related Level	38.4%

- *Patient Living Arrangements*

Live with Others (Family, Friends)	56.6%
Live Alone	43.4%

- *Discharge*

To an Acute Care Facility	61.7%
To a Residential Health Care Facility	7.8%
Patient Improved	6.9%
Patient Died	10.2%
Other (Friends, Family)	13.4%

How It Works

Certification Requirements for Providers

- Providers of services must be certified under Article 36 of the New York State Public Health Law. Detailed applications submitted to the State Department of Health describe plans for the program, including the geographic area to be served, the estimated number of visits to be provided, and the expected staffing. The application is acted upon by the appropriate health systems agency and the State Hospital Review and Planning Council, with final approval by the Commissioner of Health.

- Services regularly reimbursed by Medicaid include nursing, physical therapy, occupational therapy, speech pathology, home health aide, personal care visits, homemakers, housekeepers, medical supplies, and medical equipment and appliances and must be provided under Nursing Home Without Walls.
- Ten additional services may also be provided under the Nursing Home Without Walls program. These services are made available through a waiver from the federal government under which they have become Medicaid reimbursable. An example of a waived service is minor home improvements such as ramps and handrails. Respite service, home maintenance, and nutritional counseling are also included among the waived services.

Selection of Patients

- To be eligible for Nursing Home Without Walls patients must be medically eligible for care in a residential health care facility; their home environment must be suitable; the patient and family must want the program. The annual cost of providing care at home must not be expected to exceed 75% of the local annual Medicaid average for the appropriate level of care.
- The patient's health status and the appropriate level of care are determined by use of the DMS-1 Long Term Care Placement Form which scores the patient's physical and mental status and medical requirements. The assessment yields a score indicating the patient's required level of care. A patient residing in an area where the program is available who has been determined eligible for long-term placement must be notified of the Nursing Home Without Walls program as an alternative to institutional care by the local department of social services.
- A Home Assessment Abstract is used by the provider and the local department of social services to assess the appropriateness of the patient's home environment and types and frequency of services needed. The initial budget is based upon this information.
- If the cost is expected to be within the 75% cap on an annual basis, the services may begin.

Patient Management

- When the patient enters the program the provider must assure total management and coordination of all patient services.
- Local departments of social services share responsibility for Medicaid patients. Each patient is reassessed at least every 120 days.

Present Providers

The start-up of the program was deliberately slow and cautious to assure appropriate development. Since the nine initial providers approved in 1978 have demonstrated the success of the program the State is now encouraging its expansion. Today there are 19 programs approved in 13 counties. Additional applications are currently under consideration. Providers approved to date are:

Cattaraugus County Health Department	Cattaraugus County
Erie County Health Department	Erie County
24 Rhode Island Street Nursing Home	Erie County
Onondaga County Health Department	Onondaga County
Visiting Nurse Association of Central New York	Onondaga County
Metropolitan Jewish Geriatric Center	Kings County
Montefiore Hospital	Bronx County
St. Vincent's Hospital	New York County
Visiting Nurse Service of New York	Queens County
Eddy Geriatric Center	Rensselaer County
Rockland County Health Department	Rockland County

Jewish Home and Hospital
  for Aged   New York County

Visiting Nurse Association of
  Staten Island   Richmond County

Loretto Geriatric Center   Onondaga County

Chemung County Health
  Department   Chemung County

WK Nursing Home Company   Bronx County

St. Mary's Hospital   Kings County

Steuben County Home
  Health Agency   Steuben County

Chautauqua County Health
  Department   Chautauqua County

Endorsements

Letters from Nursing Home Without Walls patients and their families illustrate the effectiveness of the program and their satisfaction. Patients are pleased to remain in their own homes and live independently. Family members say they are alleviated of the burden of constant care for the patient, and their minds are eased since the patient receives excellent care. Health professionals attest to its cost-savings features and its patient-centered focus. Following are excerpts from some letters:

> . . . I want to tell you how happy we are with the results. In a week's time there is a vast improvement in my mother-in-law's physical and emotional condition. Her environment is more cheerful and she is looking cared for. I thank you for making her life a little better.

> Without the Nursing Home Without Walls program of your institution, there would have been no way for my parents to have been reunited, and to lead a comfortable life which is probably the exception for people of their age and physical ailment.

National Recognition

The Nursing Home Without Walls program is receiving attention across the country. Several other states are attempting to replicate the program. It served as a model for Congressional legislation—the Medicaid Community Care Act of 1980 (Waxman-Pepper) and the proposed Title XXI addition to the Social Security Act (Packwood-Bradley). The concept of Nursing Home Without Walls was included in the Federal Omnibus Reconciliation Act of 1981. Abt Associates of Cambridge, Massachusetts, conducted a three-year evaluation of the program which began in September 1979 and was funded by the Health Care Financing Administration. The report, including a case study and quantitative analysis of the data, is scheduled for publication in January 1984.

The New York City Home Care Project: A Community-Based Approach to Long-Term Care

Roberta S. Brill, MSAM

The New York City Department for the Aging is currently operating a research and demonstration project which provides maintenance level home care to the chronically ill, functionally disabled elderly. The program is funded by grants from the Federal Health Care Financing Administration and the Administration on Aging and has Medicare waivers.

The primary thrusts of the program are:

- assessment, care planning, and case management of homebound clients by an interdisciplinary team;
- coordination of existing health and social service resources; and
- supplementation with critical gap-filling services through the Medicare waivers.

For the purposes of the demonstration, the Medicare regulations have been waived which usually restrict Medicare home health coverage to those with acute, short-term skilled nursing or rehabilitative needs. The three gap-filling services, homemaker and personal care services, prescription drugs, and transportation to health and social sites, are provided to persons requiring maintenance-level care.

The target population for the Project is the Medicare recipient over 65, chronically ill, and homebound to the extent that he or she needs assistance in activities of daily living or cannot go outside without assistance. The population served are those whose incomes

Robert S. Brill is Project Director of the New York City Home Care Project, NYC Department for the Aging, New York, N.Y.

are marginally above the Medicaid level, but who cannot afford to pay for their own care.

This population was selected because of the availability of personal care services to the homebound Medicaid recipient in New York State, particularly in New York City, where the Department of Social Services operates a large-scale home attendant program. This service, which must be prescribed by a physician and supervised by a registered nurse, is a major source of community-based, long-term care for chronically ill Medicaid recipients needing maintenance-level care. This type of service is not, however, available to those older persons who are not Medicaid eligible.

There are a particularly complex variety of services for the homebound elderly in New York City which have been established by funding streams, agency history, or community initiative. Literally hundreds of agencies in the City provide home care, home health care, social services, and the supportive services. Included are meals on wheels, meals on heels, senior centers, friendly visitors, volunteer programs, telephone reassurance, homemaker services, housekeeper services, attendant services, home health aide services, and legal services, all under a variety of aegis. To complicate the situation further, services are not available uniformly in all neighborhoods throughout the City.

The complexity of the funding, the fragmentation of the programs, and the fact that each community knows its own problems best resulted in a program design that included service coordination at a community level, supplemented by some critically needed services currently not available because of funding restrictions.

To carry out the program, the New York City Department for the Aging selected four service delivery agencies to serve selected parts of New York City. Each site has the capacity to serve 100 clients at any one time. The sites have added to their staffs an assessment team of a nurse, social worker, and a physician consultant, as well as case managers and clerical staff.

The four agencies selected as Project service delivery sites include two health care agencies and two social service agencies. The health agencies are family health centers which provide ambulatory care services to both a pediatric as well as an adult population. One agency is freestanding, while the other is hospital based. Neither of the health centers had previous experience in the provision of home care services.

In contrast, the social service agencies were originally established for the sole purpose of service delivery to the elderly. Both have Title III-B programs which provide limited in-home services with funds from the New York City Department for the Aging administering the Older Americans Act.

The sites include:

- The Community Agency for Senior Citizens (CASC), a social service agency, serving all of Staten Island. Prior to the Project's inception, CASC had organized a coalition of some 35 health and social service home care and related providers to coordinate home care service delivery to the aged on the Island.
- Sunset Park Family Health Center, part of a 500-bed hospital, the Lutheran Medical Center in Brooklyn. Serving the neighborhoods of Sunset Park and Bay Ridge, the medical center is not only a major health care provider, but has taken a leadership role in such diverse areas as neighborhood development, job training, and senior citizen housing.
- Jamaica Service Program for Older Adults, a social service agency, serves a community of approximately 220,000 in Southeast Queens. This agency organized a consortium of health and social service providers to coordinate health and social services in its community.
- The Comprehensive Family Care Center of Albert Einstein College of Medicine serves a catchment area of about 235,000 in the East Central Bronx. This freestanding ambulatory care center directs much of its service to a pediatric population.

The sites are responsible for assessment, care planning, and case management, as well as the subcontracting with community agencies for the provision of waiver services. The waiver services are provided by written subcontract between the site and existing community providers such as homemaker agencies, pharmacies, and ambulette and taxi companies.

Each site follows the same process for screening, admitting, and serving clients. The assessment team makes a home visit to assess client status and service needs and to determine eligibility for the program. The assessment instrument used in our project is based on the one developed by the Georgia Health Alternatives Program, with elements from other instruments including the Access Project and the New York State nursing home assessment instrument, the

DMS-1. The interdisciplinary composition of the team reflects a commitment to the concepts that home care includes a spectrum of health and social services and that it takes an interdisciplinary team to identify the problems and to develop a plan of care for the client. If the client does not have a personal physician, the site physician makes the assessment visit.

The next step, care planning, takes into account the assessment findings and the primary care physician's evaluation. It is done by the assessment team with the involvement of the client's personal physician.

The other major component is case management. This includes arranging for services, either through another community program or directly through the Medicare waiver services. Follow-up and monitoring are major responsibilities of the case manager. They ensure that services are actually received and are meeting the client's needs. The overall status of the client is subject to continuous monitoring by the case manager and the assessment team nurse who visits at least once every three months. Formal reassessment by the team takes place every six months.

Overseeing the Project is the New York City Department for the Aging, a part of the municipal government of the City of New York, as well as the largest Area Agency on Aging in the country. It is responsible for the development of the Project, site selection, policy setting, carrying out the research and evaluation component, as well as coordination on a citywide basis. A citywide advisory committee is made up of Commissioners of the City Department of Health, Human Resources Administration, Health and Hospitals Corporation, City Planning Commission, and the local Health Systems Agency. State agencies such as the New York State Health Department and the New York State Health Planning Commission also participate, along with other experts in health care and home care.

Throughout the Project, data are being collected in some areas of critical interest to federal policymakers as well as to the Area Agency on Aging itself:

- What are the types of services needed to maintain a chronically ill, functionally disabled person at home?
- How much do they cost?
- What are the met and unmet needs in the client's physical health, mental health, housing, environment, entitlements, social services?

- Do people who receive our services fare better than those who do not? A matched comparison group of 200 people is being followed over the length of the Project to assess the Project's impact on hospitalization, nursing home placement, and utilization of health care and social services.
- What is the effect of the Project on the existing informal care system of spouses, friends, and neighbors? Do the Project's formal services provide respite for the informal supports, or do they substitute or supplement the care being given?

Program operations began in Staten Island and Brooklyn in October 1980 and in Jamaica and the Bronx in April 1981. Initial data have been collected on 504 clients and 200 in the comparison group. The preliminary data now available describe a population that is old, frail, and dependent:

- Two-thirds (68%) of the clients are over 75 years old.
- Women make up two-thirds (69%) of caseload.
- The income of the client group is marginal (66% have household incomes under $700 per month).
- Though a substantial number are Medicaid eligible, none was actually on Medicaid at the beginning of the Project.
- Fifty-five percent had been hospitalized at least once during the 12 months prior to admission to the Project.

One of the most interesting findings is related to the level of care needed by the clients, as predicted by a DMS-1 score. Scores were calculated for the first 100 clients admitted to the Project.

Nearly three-quarters of the clients have DMS-1 scores that qualify them for nursing home care. Thirty percent had scores making them eligible for Skilled Nursing Facility level care, and an additional 43% had scores making them Health Related Facility eligible.

Using another measure of dependency, the Katz scale, data indicate that the Home Care Project is serving a very disabled client group, the majority of whom are dependent in at least two basic activities of daily living.

It was somewhat unexpected that the Project would ultimately serve a population at this level of disability. The limit of 20 hours a week of homemaker/personal care service suggests that only moderately impaired older people could be maintained in the community at this level of support. However, a factor that can help explain this phenomenon is the relatively high level of informal support available to those clients. Most clients had potential family supports available. Almost half (46%) were married; two-thirds (65%) lived with others, primarily family members; 71% had at least one child and of those with children, 63% either lived with a child or were in contact with a child almost daily, while 88% had at least weekly contact. While the families of these clients, at time of assessment, were clearly carrying the major burden of care, the continued viability of their support without eventual assistance is extremely questionable. In fact, caregivers of 78% of the clients were judged by assessors to have a pressing need for respite. Therefore, Project intervention was often targeted to providing support and supplementation for family efforts, and the combined efforts of formal and informal providers enabled the Project to enroll and maintain an extremely disabled elderly population.

Future analysis of the data will explore the involvement of the caregivers for a minimum of one year after the introduction of Project services and the evolving relationship between the formal and informal caregivers. It is expected that this information will directly address the public policymakers' concern that expanded home care services will replace the care provided by families.

As the clients are followed over the course of the demonstration period, data will be collected on clients, hospitalizations, nursing home admissions, and mortality rates. Extensive data on the costs of home care services are being analyzed. When available in late 1983, the data will provide solid information for policymakers to determine the costs of expanding community-based, long-term care services.

The Erie County Coordinated Care Management Project

Maryann Bolles

Background Information

Buffalo is located in Erie County, on the shores of Lake Erie at the westernmost end of New York State. Economically, the County is dependent upon heavy industry, namely the automobile and steel industries.

The City of Buffalo is characterized by identifiable ethnic neighborhoods, which play a major role in making this a strong community. The ethnic characteristic of this community lends itself to strong familial and friendship bonds leading to an informal structure of natural support networks. Nevertheless, 26% of the elderly population live alone, and in this regard, women outnumber men by more than three to one.

Because of the major downtrend in the economy, Erie County is experiencing a projected decline in population of about 3%, but the number of its senior citizens continued to increase at a rate of 9.1% from 1970 to 1980 and will continue to increase at a rate of 17.3% from 1970 to 1985.

According to the 1980 U.S. Census reports, there are 126,176 persons 65 years of age and older in the County, of whom more than 10% are living in the rural areas. The elderly make up 12.4% of the population.

As of 1970, 30.3% of the 65 and over age group had incomes at or below the State Office for the Aging's adjusted poverty level. This percentage increases to more than 37% when considering minority elderly. Preliminary estimates of elderly with chronic limitations of a major activity of daily living show that 35% of those 65 and older in Erie County, or more than 40,000 individuals, have

Maryann Bolles is Executive Director, Coordinated Care Management Corporation, Buffalo, N.Y.

such limitations and are to some degree in need of health related supports.

Erie County closely reflects national trends in that about 5.4% of the older population are institutionalized.

Buffalo's long-term care system is fraught with problems familiar to urban communities across the country:

1. *Hospital back-up:* A survey conducted one day in 1980 found that almost 600 individuals in local hospitals were waiting for placement in long-term care institutions.
2. *A demand for nursing home beds* that exceeds the supply and that will continue to do so in the future as the elderly population increases if the present system remains unchanged.
3. *Fragmentation* and *lack of communication* among service providers.
4. A system in which the services a client receives depends more on where the person entered the system, who does the assessment and care plan, and who pays the bill rather than the needs of the client.

The result is a costly system which fails to meet the needs of the client or his family.

The Coordinated Care Management Demonstration Project

In the summer of 1979, the Robert Wood Johnson Foundation invited State Agencies on Aging to apply for grants of up to $1 million to be paid over a five-year period to demonstrate the effectiveness of integrating and coordinating at a community level the diverse array of services needed by elderly citizens with health problems. The Foundation has had success with a similar effort in the area of child health and has seen similarities in the problems involved in providing care to each group.

The approach used was the development of a community-based central coordinating unit supported by both public and voluntary sectors. The goal of the program is to organize the resources devoted to the care of the health-impaired elderly so as to improve three things:

1. access to the service system;

2. the way the system works to provide service once the individual enters the system;
3. the ability of the individual to maintain function in the environment.

The Foundation received applications from 39 states and after several elimination rounds, selected eight. The application of the Erie County Department of Senior Services was one of those selected. Other grantees are located in: Baltimore, Maryland; Cook County, Illinois; Akron, Ohio; Philadelphia, Pennsylvania; Columbia, South Carolina; Lincoln, Nebraska; and Johnson City, Tennessee.

Notice of grant award came in January 1980. I was hired as Executive Director in October 1980. Since then a small Organizational Board has expanded to 25 members, one-third of which are county officials, one-third are voluntary sector providers, and one-third are consumers. Clifford Whitman, Commissioner of the Erie County Department of Senior Services, is the President of the Board of Directors.

In addition we have established a Professional/Technical Advisory Council which includes representatives from 43 agencies involved in long-term care. We are also working with six Neighborhood Cluster Councils established by our Area Agency on Aging to facilitate program implementation. The Board/Committee Structure is interlocking. The Chairman of the Professional/Technical Advisory Council is a member of the Board of Directors and each demonstration neighborhood has a representative on the Advisory Council.

The Project is a voluntary decentralized assessment and case management coordinating unit whose prime responsibility is to help direct service agencies to provide services more effectively and efficiently and to support, through education and training, the efforts of the informal support network who provide care to the frail elderly.

We receive Robert Wood Johnson Foundation funding through a contract with the New York State Office for the Aging. State Office for the Aging staff serves on our Board of Directors and provides technical assistance, support, and monitoring to our Project. In addition, the Erie County Department of Senior Services provides substantial financial support to our effort.

The five program objectives are:

1. to identify in the community the elderly in varying states of dependency, assess their needs, and link them to available services;
2. to optimize current and available resources, and through coordination and integration, to serve an increasing number of the health-impaired elderly;
3. to work toward the development of a broad range of interventions to allow flexibility and added responsiveness in meeting the needs of the health-impaired elderly;
4. to overcome current income and eligibility restraints on services; and
5. to strengthen the natural support system.

Project Objectives

Four basic programs are planned to accomplish our objectives:

1. The Neighborhood-Based Cluster Program

We are concentrating our efforts in six neighborhoods in the City of Buffalo where Cluster Councils of health and social service providers have been formed to identify and address service coordination issues.

Coordinated Care Management Corporation staff will assist Cluster Councils:

- to clarify their role and relationship with respect to providing assessment and case management services to elderly persons in need of long-term care within their service area;
- to develop and utilize an operational definition of the target population and a priority ranking system to determine which elderly individuals are most in need of service;
- to gather patient assessment information in a uniform manner so that the basis for determining the individual's degree of impairment is the same for each agency. This will facilitate the development of a case plan based on the client's needs and desires rather than on who the assessor was or where the assessment was done;
- to establish a management information/client tracking system to monitor service delivery and to serve as a central client registry. The registry will be able to provide client assessment

and service utilization information to each participating agency, thus streamlining the process of providing appropriate services to the elderly.

2. The Informal Support Program

Recent gerontological research has shown that between 77 and 80% of services received by older people are provided by their families. In a crisis, the elderly are likely to turn to their families for help first and then to friends and neighbors. Families have been found to provide care to the point of exhaustion. They often are the link to the formal system as well.

Because, by and large, the elderly prefer to be cared for by their families and because families, to a point, are willing and able to provide needed care, it makes good sense for us to support their efforts. Coordinated Care Management Corporation (CCMC) has identified the need for training and provides information to informal service providers. The purpose of the program is to strengthen the natural support network in a neighborhood atmosphere where caregivers can share experiences and gain information. CCMC continues to provide regular monthly training programs. Specific sessions are scheduled on an ongoing basis. Topics include medication and the elderly, community resources, legal problems, personal care, and dealing with guilt and anger. Recently, the high school adult education program has offered courses of interest to the informal service providers.

3. The Hospital/Community Transition Program

This program will attempt to address what has been identified by service providers as a major problem, i.e., the need for continuity between acute care in hospitals and care in the community.

A contract has been successfully negotiated with the Erie County Health Department as have Memoranda of Understanding with the Erie County Medical Center and the Sisters of Charity Hospital. To identify elderly early on in hospitalization, a Discharge Assessment Nurse was hired in July 1982. She performs the functions of screening, assessment, care plan development, and linkage to services on all patients in the Sisters of Charity Hospital and the Erie County Medical Center who are 65 years of age or older and who reside in the demonstration areas. This collaborative effort between the hospital, community-based agencies, and the client's informal support network will smooth the transition from hospital to home thereby shortening hospital stays and reducing the likelihood of re-admission.

4. The In-Home Care Program

This program provides personal care and housekeeping services to health-impaired elderly persons who require these services to maintain themselves in the community. Our program pays for services for individuals who are not eligible for assistance through existing medical assistance programs and do not have the financial resources to pay for them or family or friends willing and able to provide care. These are the individuals who are often referred to as "falling through the cracks" of the system. Referrals for home care services come from the community and from hospitals, with priority given to functionally impaired persons residing in the demonstration areas.

In addition, CCMC staff and the Professional/Technical Advisory Council have developed the Multidisciplinary Adult Assessment, a system of uniform client assessment in use in 15 agencies in Erie County. This assessment tool allows agencies to collect comprehensive information on clients, is objective, computer-compatible, and directly relates clients' disabilities to service needs.

A two-phase process is being utilized by CCMC to maximize service coordination through uniform, comprehensive client assessment and interagency information sharing. Phase one involved the establishment of a Central Client File System. This simple, manual file system has become the very basic mechanism by which client/service information can be readily exchanged among participating agencies. Aggregate data on the elderly population residing in the demonstration areas and who have been assessed with the Multidisciplinary Adult Assessment are also accessible.

Phase two of the process investigates the development of a Management Information System that will have information processing capabilities beyond those of the Central Client File System. The Management Information System will make more comprehensive client and aggregate information available to program planners and managers in agencies that provide direct or regional planning services for the health-impaired elderly persons than is now available through the current manual Central Client File. In addition, information sharing and client tracking will be automated, offering greater responsiveness for agency personnel.

Issues

Some of the issues the project is dealing with are:

- targeting the population most in need of long-term care services;
- the development of a data base to facilitate monitoring of and planning for the long-term care system;
- strengthening the informal support system;
- matching services with needs; and
- improving communication among providers.

These issues have local and statewide implications.

Progress to Date

Now, at the beginning of our third year, we have implemented all four of our programs. A major accomplishment to date has been the development of a comprehensive assessment tool and information sharing system which is currently being used by 15 agencies.

Evaluation

The Foundation has contracted with Dr. Paul Densen and Ms. Ellen Jones of the Harvard Center for Community Health and Medical Care to evaluate all eight projects.

There will be two parts to the program evaluation; a descriptive part and a quantitative part. The descriptive part will look at:

- *Staffing*: descriptions of the director and other key personnel.
- *Significant Events*, such as:
  1. Board actions
  2. Work of Advisory Councils and Committees
  3. Significant meetings with government agencies/officials and other groups and individuals
  4. Public education events
  5. Staff and provider education events (i.e., training in use of a common assessment form)

The quantitative section will have a pre-test/post-test design. This part of the evaluation will deal with:

A. *Service Agency Profiles* at the beginning and end of the project. Some items of interest are:
   - date and type of agreement with CCMC;
   - types of service provided and licensure;
   - client eligibility;
   - caseload statistics, i.e., number of cases opened; number discharged; source of referral; number of cases by reason or place of discharge.
B. The evaluation will also look at the *functional status* and *initial source of referral* of health-impaired older people. This will provide a description of the population being served and services ordered and indicate how efficiently resources are being utilized.
C. Hospital discharge data—by place of discharge, length of stay, and admission or re-admission from institutions or the community.

Conclusion

CCMC's progress is due in large measure to the commitment of state and county government and the executives and staff of major health and social service agencies in both the private and public sector to improve the efficiency and effectiveness of the long-term care system. Long-term care coordination and integration are ideas whose time has come in Erie County.

Rensselaer County Coordinated Services: A Channeling Demonstration Project

Thomas Yandeau

The National Long Term Care Channeling Demonstration Project grew out of the necessity to create the prototype for a comprehensive integrated service delivery system. After years of "lip service" to the barriers to effective and efficient service delivery to the elderly, human service professionals, nationwide, have been given the opportunity to test many of their hypotheses and help create a policy that will allow for the necessary service delivery system changes. In a nation of shrinking resources, this task is being undertaken earnestly and with the realization that this might be the last effort at creating a positive policy regarding long-term care for the elderly.

The Channeling Project is funded jointly by the Administration on Aging (AoA) and the Health Care Financing Administration (HCFA) under the direction of the Assistant Secretary for Planning and Evaluation (ASPE). This is a research program designed to test the effectiveness and efficiency of case management in organizing and delivering services and controlling costs. "Channeling" refers to a case management approach to organizing and delivering community-based health and social services to chronically impaired elderly.

The National Program included twelve local sites in the United States. Since New York State was interested in participating in the National Program, site proposals were sought from the various county human service agencies statewide. Upon reviewing this request, the Rensselaer County Department for the Aging identified this as a program which might begin to meet some of the long-term

Thomas Yandeau is Coordinator of Aging Services, Rensselaer County Department for the Aging, Troy, N.Y.

care needs that the Aging Department had identified in Rensselaer County.

Rensselaer County had identified a strong need for a systems change through the direct line observations of caseworkers, information and referral staff, and public health nurses. Also, in 1978, the National Association of Counties Research Foundation selected Rensselaer County as one of six locations throughout the country to do a comprehensive needs assessment over a 20-year period to determine the needs of Rensselaer County by the year 2000. The completed needs analysis strongly pointed out the need for a comprehensive, coordinated service delivery system for long-term care. During the Spring and Summer of 1979, after the Long Term Plan had been released, a local foundation for the elderly began working with Rensselaer County to attempt to establish a program of uniform case management, assessment, and authorization of services. The program, as outlined, strongly resembled the Department of Health and Human Services' (DHHS) proposed Channeling Project. A decision was then made by the County to answer the Request for Proposal and pursue the establishment of such a program.

When the Department for the Aging submitted its first three-page proposal, there was no premonition of what sort of work and involvement was to ensue. The Summer of 1980 saw several rewrites, more detailed submissions, and intensive planning on this project. As a result, Rensselaer County became one of three finalists in New York State that would be included in New York's submission to DHHS. In September, the announcement was made that New York State had been selected as one of twelve locations across the country to sponsor a Long Term Care Channeling Demonstration Project. However, the County's application process was not over yet. One more rewrite of the County's draft submission resulted in a 210-page document spelling out exactly what was planned and how the County planned to do it. In January 1981, it was announced that Rensselaer County had been chosen as the site for New York's Long Term Care Channeling Demonstration Project, with an anticipated operational budget of $1.5 million over a five-year period.

Since that announcement, there have been many changes in the National Channeling Program. Rescission Committee funding cuts necessitated that the original five-year funding period be decreased to four years. Additionally, the total number of sites across the country was decreased from 12 sites to 10. Research concerns precipitated a change in target population. The original target population emphasized persons 65 years of age and older, but with the ability to serve an age range of 18 to 64 years. Now, the target population is limited to persons 65 years of age and over.

Through the utilization of a telephone screening interview, the Project attempts to identify appropriate potential participants. Criteria for participation are:

1. two moderate ADL impairments or three severe IADL impairments,
2. two unmet service needs, or fragile informal support system,
3. willingness to participate,
4. Rensselaer County resident,
5. age 65 or over.

These criteria are an attempt to operationalize the target population description which identifies potential clients as those persons over 65 years of age who are at risk of institutionalization.

After screening, appropriate potential participants will be randomized into control and treatment groups. The treatment group is the Channeling Project's caseload. As a research project, when full caseload is reached, there will be 200 clients in Channeling's caseload and an additional 200 project participants in the control group.

Mathematica Policy Research (MPR) is responsible for maintenance of the control group and collecting all data required from the control group. Channeling staff will conduct the baseline assessment with clients and reassess clients every six months. MPR will conduct research interviews in between reassessments.

The Project initiated services in June 1982, and full caseload should have been attained by June 1983. This full caseload will be maintained for 18 months. At the completion of 18 months at full caseload, a six-month phase-out will be undertaken.

Prior to initiation of services, staff were hired and trained. As a unit of the Department for Aging, the Project Director answers directly to the Commissioner of Aging. This unit will consist of 8 professional staff (senior case manager, research analyst, one public health nurse, four case managers, and one screener), in addition to five ancillary staff. The screener will be responsible for conducting the comprehensive screen to determine appropriateness for the Project. Those potential participants determined appropriate and randomized into the treatment group will receive a comprehensive assessment by a case manager. A care plan will be developed from the assessment by the case manager in consultation with the public health nurse. After reviewing the care plan with the client and getting the client's written approval, the case manager will initiate service delivery.

After developing this basic client flow, DHHS requested Rensselaer County to become one of five "complex model" sites. As a complex model, a site has a much stronger intervention in the community. The increased strength of intervention results from increased authority over service and Medicare waivers. The Medicare Waivers gave a package of services to Medicare-eligible clients which are not now reimbursable under Medicare. This service package consists of adult day care, homemaker/personal care, mental health, respite, transportation, home-delivered meals, housing assistance, and home health services. Some clients will pay a small share of their costs.

Additionally, as a complex model, a site has the authority to authorize the amount, scope, and duration of services under Medicaid and Medicare. Moreover, funds from Title III and Community Service for the Elderly (CSE) have been earmarked for use by the site.

Complex model sites will have an agency cap with flexibility for individual client costs. This agency cap will be generated by funds pooled from Title III, Title XIX, CSE, and Medicare-waivered dollars.

There have been interesting experiences which resulted from seeking to participate in the National Project. First, the County legislature was very hesitant to accept money in light of federal cutbacks. The primary questions were: "would the funding be cut" and "would the County be expected to continue the program using county dollars, in spite of the fact that federal dollars had been withdrawn?" A second, and more important issue was the Project's emphasis on research and the subsequent control for standardization. Among concerns raised were:

1. local determination of operation procedures;
2. slowness of developing the materials at the federal level;
3. the length of the screening and assessment forms;
4. randomization in control groups, "not everyone referred and appropriate will receive service, creating a local moral issue";

5. complicated screening and intake procedures because of the research aspect.

In order to deal with such issues, the Project established an Advisory Board in June of 1980, consisting of all local health care providers and consumers. This was created prior to any commitment to the Project, under the assumption that even if the County did not receive project funding, it would try to initiate the concept of channeling locally. The Board has worked closely with staff on various aspects of the Project.

Initially there were the anticipated turf problems. Providers expressed the feeling that case management was already being done in Rensselaer County, and, in general, displayed skepticism about federal grant programs and demonstration projects. As Advisory Board involvement has matured, there has been a tremendous increase of support and productivity. Among other major areas of local concern, was concern about increased Medicaid expenditures as a result of the program. Local public officials have worried that the Project will increase the number of elderly in the County identified as Medicaid eligible. However, it is anticipated that decreased institutionalization rates and the use of Medicare waivers will offset this problem.

Such concerns naturally have statewide implications. State agencies such as the Office of Health Systems Management (OHSM), the Department of Social Services (DSS), and the State Office for the Aging (SOFA) have had to determine which state regulations can be amended, and how much authority and flexibility will be given to the Project.

The impact of the Channeling Project will be felt nationwide, as well as statewide and countywide. Project results will be used to shape national long-term care policy. Thus, evaluation of the Project and the research is of utmost importance. The evaluation process will be conducted in three ways:

1. A service audit and program review will be conducted by the State.
2. As a national research project, there will be continual monitoring by a federal subcontractor of all research aspects and components.
3. There will be ongoing, continual self-evaluation of the Project, its goals, and its effectiveness.

With the results and data from the Project and its evaluation, the National Long Term Care Demonstration will address several policy questions:

1. Does channeling reduce institutionalization and increase the utilization of community and informal health and social services by clients?
2. Does channeling reduce the public costs of long-term care; how does it affect private expenditures for services; what are the costs of channeling itself; and what determines these costs?
3. Does channeling result in reduced functional deterioration, improved quality of life (using both objective and subjective measures), and lower mortality for channeling clients as compared to the control group?
4. How does channeling affect the personal and financial burden of care placed on families, and the maintenance of family supports?
5. Does channeling alter the mix of service supplied by particular types of providers, the referral patterns among providers, and the amount or charge for services supplied in community or institutional settings?
6. What types of individuals (categorized by age, sex, income, type of impairment, etc.) participate in channeling, and what determines their participation?
7. Does the channeling intervention and variations of it strengthen the capacity of the long-term care system to meet client needs in an efficient and effective manner, and what approaches to implementing channeling would be most effective for national replication?
8. Is channeling a cost-effective, long-term care policy intervention, and is it relatively more cost effective for certain types of interventions and certain subgroups of the target population?

The Rensselaer County Department for the Aging is proud to be participating in this National Research Project. It is hoped that the Project will not only initiate sound federal policy, but will also affect state and county long-term care policy. But most important, in participating, the Project will provide 200 of the County's frail elderly with comprehensive, integrated, long-term care services in order to maintain them within their homes.

Metropolitan Jewish Geriatric Center: From Multi-Level Long-Term Care Institution to Social/Health Maintenance Organization

Dennis L. Kodner

Long-term care is the domain concerned with diminished capacity for self-care resulting from disabling physical and/or mental conditions. While long-term care may be aimed in part at rehabilitation, its main thrust is to prevent or delay further breakdowns in functioning and to maintain a satisfactory quality of life. A prime consideration in meeting the long-term care needs of the elderly and chronically impaired population is the integration of health-related care with those social, psychological, and environmental supports that may improve a person's coping ability as well as provide adequate solutions to problems of everyday life.

Policymakers, planners, and professionals almost universally agree that the current patch quilt of services and funding in the health and human service sectors cannot accomplish these long-term care objectives. Needless to say, resolving this problem is a task of considerable urgency.

As an alternative to today's fragmented, costly, and inappropriate long-term care non-system, efforts are underway on the federal, state, and local levels to develop comprehensive, coordinated systems which provide access to a broad array of health and social care in the least restrictive and most cost-effective environments.

Nursing homes are central to the long-term care problem and

Dennis L. Kodner is General Director, Elderplan, Inc. At the time of this presentation, Mr. Kodner was Director of Planning & Community Services at Metropolitan Jewish Geriatric Center. Elderplan, Inc. is the corporate entity sponsored by the Center to operate the Social/Health Maintenance Organization demonstration project.

have been associated, more often than not, with inappropriate use and high cost on the one hand, and negativism on the other. As a result, long-term care facilities have traditionally been excluded from the mainstream of health and human services for the elderly. However, since the late 1970s, they have emerged as a vital part of efforts to reform the long-term care system in many communities throughout the country and are now recognized as a potential resource to initiate, coordinate, and deliver comprehensive health services for older adults.

The geriatric center, if designated properly, can become the flexible base for community services within the context of differing living arrangements. Because of its strategic location as the most intensive cluster of services at the end of the long-term care continuum, the geriatric center can expand and redirect existing staff and institutional programs to provide care outside its four walls. This could save the substantial costs of setting up a new network of non-institutional services, provide an easy link between points on the service array, offer a single focal point for local accountability, and assure that needed care is indeed provided when and where needed.

A number of attempts have been made in the past to develop multi-level or campus-type complexes in which a single administrative unit offers a wide range of services including skilled nursing and intermediate care, protective living arrangements, adult daycare, meals programs, mental health and counseling services, and limited in-home care. These programs have demonstrated the willingness and capability of long-term care institutions to meet the multiple needs of the aged and to become "geriatric centers" in the fullest sense of the word. Metropolitan Jewish Geriatric Center, a large, multi-level facility, has gone way beyond this approach to outreach programming and is in the process of transforming itself into a gerontological health center designed to serve the increasing needs of well and impaired older persons for both acute and chronic care. This unique model has implications for long-term care system reform and cost-control activities as well as ongoing efforts to define, evaluate, and improve the quality of long-term care.

Established in 1907, Metropolitan Jewish Geriatric Center (MJGC) is a 915-bed voluntary, non-profit, long-term care institution. The Center, which is affiliated with the Federation of Jewish Philanthropies of New York and is accredited by the Joint Commission on Accreditation of Hospitals, is located in an area of New York City with one of the nation's largest elderly populations. In recent years, Metropolitan has developed a large number of innovative community services under its own roof. The facility's comprehensive, interdisciplinary philosophy is in keeping with the belief that the current health system for the elderly is piecemeal, institutionally biased, over-medicalized, and wasteful in both financial and human terms. The Center's "umbrella" approach provides ready access to progressive patient care in either direction. In this way, patients are hopefully diverted from unnecessary or unwanted institutional care, thus enabling them to carry on their present life-style in the community. In addition, temporary or permanent admission to the nursing home is assured when it is either desired or warranted.

Since 1977, Metropolitan Jewish Geriatric Center has developed a large number of outreach programs designed to meet the multiple needs of the elderly. They include a Day Hospital, Medicaid-waived Long Term Home Health Care Program, State-Designated Hospice Demonstration Project, Respite Service, Emergency Alarm Response System, and Transportation for the Elderly and Handicapped. The Center was recently designated by the University Health Policy Consortium at Brandeis University's Heller Graduate School of Social Welfare—acting as the agent of the U.S. Health Care Financing Administration—as the first site in a multi-size national demonstration of the Social/Health Maintenance Organization (S/HMO).

DESCRIPTION OF CURRENT OUTREACH EFFORTS

The Day Hospital

Adult day health care, also known as day hospital care and by a variety of other terms, is one of the most flexible ways of organizing health, social, and supportive services to meet the needs of older people and their families for long-term care, health maintenance, and psychosocial services to the high-risk elderly in order to shorten a hospital or nursing home stay or prevent or delay institutional placement.

The Day Hospital at MJGC opened its doors in 1977 and was the Center's first outreach program. It provides one-stop medical and nursing care, rehabilitation, social services, recreational activities, and hot meals, as well as round-trip transportation to 50 participants. Depending on individual needs, participants attend six hours daily, several days per week.

Our experience with the Day Hospital has been quite positive. It helps maintain older persons in their own homes, makes their lives more meaningful and productive, provides relief and support to their families, and prevents and forestalls their premature institutionalization.

"Nursing Home Without Walls"

The realities of fragmented home care funding and administration on the local, state, and national levels prevent community-based care from being a truly effective deterrent to institutionalization.

One frequently proposed solution to this problem is to establish within each community a single agency that directly provides all in-home services. Staff would be responsible for identifying the population-at-risk, making an interdisciplinary assessment of client needs, and then developing a comprehensive plan of care. Patients would have to deal with one agency, which would provide most, if not all, of the needed services available in the community. New York's "Nursing Home Without Walls" is one such innovative model which has attracted nationwide attention.

As a result of Metropolitan's success with the Day Hospital, the Center became one of the original nine Long Term Home Health Care Programs to participate in the "Nursing Home Without Walls" pilot project. It began operations in 1979 and is considered one of the state's most successful demonstration sites. The program's current certified capacity is 300 clients.

Analysis of demographic characteristics of the 511 unduplicated patients served by MJGC since May of 1979 indicates that the average person qualified for SNF care is female, age 77, has a major circulatory problem, lives with relatives, was referred to the program from a community agency, and is most frequently discharged to the hospital. Early evaluation findings seem to confirm the view that MJGC's caseload is one of the most seriously impaired in the entire statewide "Nursing Home Without Walls" program.

Preliminary cost data collected by the Center suggest that the facility's LTHHCP is 47% less costly than the equivalent level of HRF and SNF care. In addition to these major savings, there is evidence of postponed hospital and nursing home use, improved quality of life, and strong consumer satisfaction with the program.

Hospice Care

There is considerable professional and grassroots interest in providing comfort care to terminally ill patients and their families. Called "hospice," such coordinated physical, emotional, and spiritual support is seen as a means of improving the quality of remaining life for the dying and as a way to reintegrate survivors into the community of living.

The development of hospice in the United States has been extremely individualized. There are many approaches, each differing in terms of setting, services, staffing, and finances. Hospice can be organized by a hospital, nursing home, freestanding facility, or home health agency. Needless to say, hospice is considered entirely compatible with the Center's philosophy and patient care system.

Metropolitan began studying the feasibility of establishing a hospice in late 1978. The Center filed an application with the State Department of Health in June 1979 requesting designation as a hospice demonstration project as part of the state's pilot program to test the concept with the intent of eventual licensure. The hospice was designated as one of 14 programs statewide in September and began operations in January 1980.

The Brooklyn Hospice, as the Center's program is called, is a coordinated program of in-home, outpatient, and institutional care. It also includes patient transportation, "aftercare" for bereaved family members, and consultation and education services.

The hospice program's focus on in-home and outpatient care with the inpatient service as back-up is made possible by the institution's patient care continuum. Responsibility for home care is lodged in the Long Term Home Health Care Program. Outpatient care is provided by the Day Hospital. Hospice patients who require inpatient palliation are placed in the Skilled Nursing Facility's Maximum Care Unit. When appropriate, other home health nursing agencies, nursing homes, and hospitals are utilized.

The Brooklyn Hospice represents a major effort by a multi-level geriatric center to develop a supportive program for the dying using the facility's extensive inpatient and community resources as the basic building blocks. The program has already served several hundred patients and families since its inception. However, even though the project has demonstration status, it has experienced considerable financial difficulties which must be overcome in order to achieve stability.

Respite Service

Practical experience in working with the institutional elderly as well as the professional literature confirm that breakdowns in the informal support system are the primary cause of admissions to the nursing home. Respite care, an idea developed in Scandinavia and Britain, provides an incentive to care for frail elderly persons in the home by giving temporary physical and psychological relief to spouses, adult children, and other family caregivers.

Respite can be provided at home through a homemaker/home health aide agency or in an institutional setting. Metropolitan's "Visiting Resident" program provides temporary institutional care for six weeks or less to persons who are otherwise eligible for placement in a long-term care facility. The present respite service consists of four beds in the facility's Health Related Facility unit. Persons may be admitted directly from the Center's Long Term Home Health Care Program, Day Hospital, Hospice, or the community.

The "Visiting Resident" program, initiated in mid-1981, has already served 17 persons. Because of growing demand for respite care in the community, consideration is being given to extending the project to include respite beds in the skilled nursing pavilion. The project, which is part of a larger multi-site demonstration sponsored by the New York Association of Homes for the Aging, will be evaluated in terms of cost, consumer satisfaction, and delayed institutionalization.

Electronic Monitoring

While some chronically impaired elderly need extensive home care services, others only require minimal monitoring to ensure their well-being and independent living. Monitoring exists in the form of friendly visiting, daily telephone calls, and more passive approaches like electronic alert systems.

The Center now operates an Emergency Alarm Response System (EARS) which provides an electronic link between the client's home and an around-the-clock receiving station.

The system, which has already been extensively tested under a DHHS grant, has the potential of reducing the need for long-term health care. It also makes elderly clients more secure about living alone and confident about reaching a health facility or community agency in an emergency.

Clients in the Center's various outreach programs are eligible for EARS, as are community residents. Currently there are 135 persons linked to the system; it will be expanded to 250 subscribers in the near future.

AN OVERVIEW OF THE MJGC EXPERIENCE

There are many obstacles that must be overcome in order to develop an integrated long-term care system, especially when using the multi-level geriatric center as the resource base. What happens in the future will depend on local politics, professional and organizational attitudes, and national and state policies. The following is a brief list of some of the more important problems that Metropolitan has faced in providing holistic care for older people:

1. Disjointed administration of multiple federal, state, and local programs, differing funding arrangements, and the varying scopes of benefits and eligibility requirements make it difficult to fit all the long-term care pieces together in a comprehensive delivery system.
2. "Turf" issues represent a major challenge to any provider wishing to play a key role in reforming the long-term care system. This is especially relevant to long-term care institutions which are viewed in a very narrow sense by other health and human service agencies serving the elderly in the community.
3. Geriatric centers involved in developing and operating community-based programs will have a difficult time in overcoming widespread negative stereotypes and in gaining broad-based, local acceptance.
4. Existing reimbursement does not provide adequate funding of non-institutional services, especially with regard to needed planning and outreach efforts.
5. The operation of community services by multi-level, long-term care institutions exerts a strain on the facility's resources, management capabilities, and leadership abilities. This can force institutions into an ongoing conflict over scarce resources between the program needs of residents/inpatients and community clients.

Despite these formidable problems, MJGC's experience has been overwhelmingly positive. The traditional image of the facility as an "old age home" has given way to local and national recognition as a truly comprehensive geriatric center and an enhanced reputation as an innovator in the fields of aging and long-term care. Integration between Metropolitan and the surrounding communities has materialized, and there is now the strong feeling among Board members, administration, staff, clients, and their families that we are doing all we can to provide the most appropriate care and support of the elderly population.

PRE-PAID SOCIAL/HEALTH CARE: A NEW DIRECTION

Although the Center has made major strides in expanding the institution's resources into the community for the benefit of older people living at home, particularly those with disabling conditions, the comprehensive service system is far from complete. Because decreased federal and state spending threatens the quality of care for elderly persons, the Center is exploring new ways to organize, deliver, and finance gerontological health services for both the well and impaired aged populations. As was noted above, Metropolitan was recently designated by the University Health Policy Consortium at Brandeis University's Heller School—HCFA's national agent— as the nation's first Social/Health Maintenance Organization (S/HMO). Collaborating in the project is Cornell University's Medical College Division of Geriatrics and Gerontology. Called Elderplan, the S/HMO would provide a full range of acute and long-term care services in institutional and community settings using a capitated financing method in which a specified amount of Medicare and Medicaid funds and direct consumer payments would be provided to the central organization for an enrolled population. Like the Health Maintenance Organization model, the S/HMO would be "at risk" for costs above the capitated amount.

In order to keep costs under tight control, the S/HMO would provide comprehensive assessment and case management services, provide many direct services on its own, and contract with provider agencies in the community. It will also emphasize programs which prevent further functional decline and attempt to substitute lower cost in-home and community-based services in lieu of the hospital or nursing home.

Planning and development efforts have been ongoing since January 1982 with principal funding from the John A. Hartford Foundation. Plans call for the enrollment of 4,000 older persons starting in June 1983. Targeted marketing activities will be aimed at attracting a representative mix of elderly, including about 18% of the membership falling into the moderately and extremely impaired categories and some 21% of the total eligible for Medicaid.

As this organizational option is pursued, Metropolitan Jewish Geriatric Center will gradually evolve from a geriatric center with numerous levels and settings of care into a comprehensive gerontological health system with a long-term care institution as one of its many programs and facilities.

Part III

KEY ISSUES

Introduction to Part III

In Part II, seven coordinated long-term care service programs developed in New York State under varying sponsors and funding streams were described. Despite their differences, all of these programs shared the following four areas of concern and interest:

1. system organization,
2. case management,
3. cost effectiveness,
4. evaluation and assessment.

These four areas are discussed in Part III. McNally is concerned about financial limitations and how they will affect system organization. Green and Ashton deal with different approaches to case management. Kodner is concerned with whether it is too soon to determine cost effectiveness of community-based, long-term care programs. And Gurland, Bennett, and Wilder express a view similar to Kodner's noting that it may be too soon to evaluate the impact of community-based, long-term care programs since there are so few of them. It is possible that they may supplement rather than be substitutes for institutions. This may lead both to ambiguous research results as well as increased costs at this time.

Despite obvious differences in assessments used, research design, program elements, as well as sponsors and funders, it is the similar and shared concerns that are described in Part III.

Issues in System Organization and Development of Community-Based, Long-Term Care Services: Utilization, Access, Assessment, and Gatekeeping

Leonard McNally

Introduction

A number of issues of how best to organize community-based, long-term care services are discussed in the major portion of this chapter. While it seems desirable to have demonstration programs in the state, there is some concern about whether the state will be able to utilize the results obtained from these demonstrations throughout the state.

Major issues addressed are: (1) fiscal management, (2) gatekeeping authority, and (3) assessment. Who should provide services and where they should best be provided are questions asked.

These questions arise against a background of dwindling resources; certainly, there will be no more money available in the future for delivering services than there is at present. It is anticipated that there are going to be caps and there are going to be cutbacks. Somehow we have to determine how the services are going to be delivered with less money and, also, we have to develop the ability to make decisions on where people can receive services in the most cost-effective manner. Thus, as the population increases, more people should be able to get less expensive services. Effective organization may be the key to achieving this.

Leonard McNally is Long Term Care Planner, Health Systems Agency of New York City.

Ideas for this paper were also contributed by the following panel members: Roberta Brill, Gerald Eggert, and Robert O'Connell.

Role of Model Programs for Planning

Those of us responsible for developing a statewide plan for services in the future require knowledge of what the model assessments, referrals, and programs are going to do to alter in any way the need for services. It is hoped that community-based, coordinated service systems for the delivery of long-term care will reduce the need for nursing home care. It seems that in any kind of home care project, 70% of home care clients turn out to have been eligible for nursing homes. One explanation for this figure is that perhaps on a DMS-1* form everyone would be eligible for a nursing home. But what we do not know from this figure is whether or not all of those who are eligible would have gone to a nursing home. The reasons that people go to a nursing home are poorly understood and unfortunately all the formulas that we start using are based on past utilization experience. Thus, it is difficult to determine how new programs are going to modify past utilization. In developing a new state formula for nursing-home bed need, there is a general determination of long-term health care need. But in developing this formula the new community-based programs are not included. It should be possible to determine bed need and then subtract out the number of clients in the home health care programs.

Planning bodies should take the results of these demonstration projects into consideration and build them into the planning process. The Health Planning Commission (HPC) has been involved in some of the demonstration projects described in Part II above more than others.

In long-term and health care the HPC is involved in the certificate of need program. However, the HPC is not involved in an Article 36 state-certified program conducted by New York City's Department for the Aging because there was never a certificate of need required. Thus, HPC only served in an advisory capacity and reviewed their first grant proposal. The HPC is still waiting to be able to feed in some concrete results from the demonstration projects and to be able to put them into a formulation that will stand up to legal scrutiny. This is needed because one cannot tell a nursing home operator he cannot have another nursing home without fearing a potential suit. And the experience in the courts is that the operator

---

*DMS-1 is a standard form for documentation of medical status provided by the New York State Department of Health to be used for long-term care placement.

usually wins and that the state and the regulatory body usually lose. Thus for each theoretical plan that sounds good, one has to figure out how it is going to stand up in court.

Sometimes, however, the results shown by the data may backfire. Monroe County (see Part II) has perhaps the best and the longest running program for keeping people out of nursing homes, but it also has the most nursing homes in the state. This sort of finding makes it very confusing to deal with the data. Despite this sort of confusion, the Health Planning Commission is interested in trying to put the results into a concrete supportable methodology for determining long-term care needs at various levels of care. There is no satisfactory method for determining the need for home care any more than for nursing home care. But nursing homes usually win because they have been around a lot longer. There has never been any major support for home care. Perhaps after the demonstration results are all in we will have some better idea of how many slots or how many programs are needed in home care, where they should be, and what kinds of services they should contain.

Home Care Versus Nursing Home Care

The 709.3 need methodology refers to that part of the hospital code that determines need for residential health care facilities which is the hospital code term for skilled nursing (SNF) and health related (HRF) facilities. New York State is concerned that an indefinite amount of nursing home care may not be available because in New York State about 75% to 80% of the costs of nursing homes are borne by the Medicaid program. In New York City, the costs are even higher; about 93% of the nursing home costs are borne by Medicaid. Thus, every nursing home that the state allows to be built has to be paid for by the state, a situation quite unique to the nursing home industry as far as building medical facilities in actual concrete is concerned. Because of this, no one is satisfied with the existing determination of needs methodology because if there is this much utilization today and there are going to be many more people in the old age group tomorrow, costs will go up if and when we build any more beds. Straight line methodology with some modifications based on what are called reasonable use ranges were developed in the late '60s in the Rochester area where almost all the long-term care demonstration work in the state has ever been done. However, there was a great deal of dissatisfaction with that. Currently, a new formulation is developing which takes many more factors into consideration. Whether or not this new formulation process is done on any stronger methodological basis is not known. One of the things considered now is that the number of nursing home beds needed will be based on a calculation which subtracts out long-term home care; 5% to 8% of the nursing homes that would have been needed by 1985 will be subtracted out and the funds will be allocated for long-term home care. That issue is quite controversial and has not been adopted yet but that is what is on the drafting table.

Long-term health care is expanding right now, but the rate has slowed down. By 1985, it will be interesting to see if there will be many providers, particularly considering the fact that to date the typical provider has been a rather well endowed voluntary medical provider. Because of the questionable availability of funds, not many groups are interested in offering long-term health care programs. It will be very interesting to see if there will be new providers that do not have quite as much money that are interested after the new formula is put into use.

We know very well that long-term care can be offered cheaply, and it can be done very well if you look at the traditional home attendant program experience. It is a good program and can be offered to a lot of people.

Throughout the state, e.g., Rochester and Syracuse, many have tried to determine how you would evaluate traditional home care. In New York City in 1980, about 100,000 people received home care, about 25,000 of those from the home attendant program. We are pretty sure that a large number of the home attendant clients, particularly the ones receiving 24-hour attendant service, would have been in a nursing home or would have had to go to a nursing home if the program had not been there. However, we do not know how many potential clients there are. Did it reach all of them? Did it reach 10%, 20%, or all of the 24 hour ones? We don't know. One thing we know is that the program does not have data to help us to make an assessment.

Traditional home care services care for the majority. The Visiting Nurse Service (VNS) delivers the traditional programs, and these are hospital-based programs. The reasons for using the VNS is that there is a state contract with the VNS and, thus, it delivers most of the service. We suspect that at least 50% of those patients served by the VNS are not candidates for nursing homes. Most are getting short-term, post hospital rehabilitative-type home care. They will go on the program and will be off the program in 50 days. Thus, we do not want to say that VNS is relieving the need for nursing homes. What percent of the caseload is relieving the need is not known. It is not surprising that New York City with the best home care system in the country has also been utilizing more nursing homes than any place else. This does not seem to be a coincidence; there may be an interrelationship in that fact. But how can it be put into a formula representing a numerical interrelationship? But a formula has to be put into the hospital code; it will have to have numbers that can be derived from it and it will have to be supportable legally. In short we do not know how to feed traditional home care into the formula.

The traditional home attendant program must be fitted into the equation. New York City's Home Attendant program for better or for worse is serving an awful lot of people, probably some well and some very poorly. We need to determine what we are going to be willing to accept. While it is fine to conduct all these demonstrations described above, one needs to point out that the home attendant program is serving tens of thousands of people in New York City.

Now how do we decide who gets the traditional program, who gets the Lombardi nursing home without walls program, and who gets the personal care program? Thus far, there seems little on which to base a decision. However, in a way it already has been decided because we can only do what we can afford and that is a decision that is going to be out of our control. While there are pretty good assessment tools that can help us decide, eligibility formulations are chiefly used.

Reimbursement for Home Care as a Limiting Factor

Medicaid is not a very good national reimbursement source for home care, though in New York State Medicaid is a fairly good source. Seventy-five percent of all Medicaid home care in the country is used in New York State, and about 75% of that is used in New York City. Medicaid in most states is less likely to reimburse for home care than Medicare. How to give a comprehensive home care program to a non-Medicaid client is a problem in New York. There is going to be a cap on costs, and it will be necessary to determine within that cap which service is the most appropriate. At this point, many of us think that we can give more home care to more people for the same amount of dollars it would take to build a small number of nursing homes. But this seems highly unlikely in the future.

In 1979 the state came up with what it was going to call a capital capitation; it would approve only x amount of new construction. This was primarily aimed at nursing homes and hospitals and meant that in New York State one would allow x amount of money to be spent on capital construction and no more. Thus, money would have to be allocated for what we need the most. Well, as you can imagine, that program was never instituted. The controversy over such programs is very real, but that is what we are going to need in the next few years. The idea about the minimum standard in a nursing home is interesting. Within the state, consumer groups push for maximum standards. The hospital and state councils have deferred action on the approval of a new nursing home on Long Island not because nursing homes are not needed but because it would be the Cadillac of nursing homes. It would have everything. The state has neither disapproved nor approved. They have done nothing and are asking: Do we disapprove? Do we approve contingent on their cutting $50 million out of the project so that it is the basic nursing home and not a Cadillac? Can the state make such a demand? The home happens to be a division of Metropolitan Jewish Geriatric Center so we are dealing with a group that has the money to build the Cadillac: they can get loans, they can build it at 18%, and they can get a conventional mortgage because it is a relatively wealthy provider. There's a temptation to go out on the market, get the mortgage, build the place and then the state has to pay it back.

Competition

One cannot ignore the competitive model. In order to have optimal organization without having a monopoly means that you allow an element of competition which enables you to be more efficient. One idea is to establish capitalization rates and let people bid on running the organization. Let's say you have to put up a bond for $250,000, which is your risk capital, that is, how much you want to lose. Then you register that amount as a bank does. That amount is the bottom line. Then, the state or federal government says that last year we paid $3,000 a year for long-term care clients. That is the bottom line; if you go over $3,000 a year, then you start eating into your $250,000 capital. But if you provide services for under $3,000 then the government could share the risk. Thus, the amount of money you saved can go into providing new services. You increase your assets by, say, putting only half of your money into the pool while the government pays the other half. Organizations should compete with each other to see who can provide a certain minimal level of service more cheaply.

The issue of private pay always surfaces. Right now basically long-term care in New York State means the state pays. I think what we have to do is start to rethink the issue of private pay and determine when the state needs to take over payment. They are getting back to private pay for long-term care in some states. In some states, there are preadmission screening programs to determine if clients will be eligible for Medicaid in three months. This is not done in New York. While it is one thing to have 50 programs in 50 states, it is quite another to have 50 programs in one state and it is hard to see how we are going to avoid having 50 programs in New York State as things stand now.

If all of a sudden the state gets comparable services and some run 10% less than the others, the state should support the cheaper ones. The fiscal manager will determine how to get the best return for the money invested. Such a competitive system will provide a very quick levelling approach, especially in the home care field. The private pay client might get a minimum benefit. If they want to go above it on an individual private pay basis they should be able to pay for it. But the private pay client should not have to be enrolled in Medicaid to get some of its benefits. Philosophically we may all be committed to having the voluntary and the non-profit homes provide long-term care. Unfortunately, the experience in the home health field has been that even the largest voluntary agency cannot attract excellent business expertise into it because there is not enough money to pay them or lure them.

Between the home care agency and the nursing home, it ought to be possible to determine who can provide a certain minimum amount of care for a specified amount of money. In New York State we have 2.1 million people over the age of 65, with 13% or 273,000 potentially in need of long-term care. Five to eight thousand people could be assigned to a long-term care unit, each one of which is managed independently. Some would manage better than others and might get returns on their investments. The state should help them perhaps by renegotiating their annual rate. That might be the major role to be played by the state. Basically you need some good fiscal managers. Many groups are going to break their budget in the first two months. Then they will have 50 elderly people enrolled in a program and will have spent all their money. Then what will they do; they are going to be running to the state saying we have nobody to give them service. The state is going to have to bail them out and that is going to happen in at least half the programs set up. What do you do if they run out of money in two months? At least the first half million should be their own money.

The Role of the State in Planning

Some state agencies are determined to let local communities plan and do everything for themselves. There will be a few local volunteers to help medical providers and they will come up with some unworkable concepts. This is because many people do not want big agencies or corporations to tell them where their mothers should go. They would prefer to have a little church group make such decisions. But this can result in great losses of money. There is a perfect example of this in New York State in the past. Article 28 of the nursing home code allowed homes to be built with no cash. You just needed to have land; that was cash. In other words, the land was worth 5% of the cost of the project. One of the places built on these terms is in serious financial trouble now. At this point, the state will no longer allow anybody to come up with a piece of land and say it is 5% of the cost of the project so we will build. At this point the state expects you to come up with 15%. Moreover you can no longer come up with $1.5 million in your pocket to design a $10 million program.

Gatekeeping Authority

The key to providing services less expensively is gatekeeping authority. Whoever is the gatekeeper needs to be able to determine who is eligible for nursing homes. What is keeping the utilization rate of nursing home beds down today is the fact that there are no beds available. In point of fact the DMS-1 assessment form may well be doing the state more harm than good. It was probably devised to tell people what level of care they were eligible for, as well as to keep people out of nursing homes. But that has been reversed and now it has insured them of the right to go into nursing homes. Thus, assessment by itself is not gatekeeping and should not be used to determine level of care needed or what facility is needed.

Assessment

Assessment is a key to gatekeeping. However, assessment instruments are not making management decisions. They give one the data upon which to exercise professional judgment about services needed. But whether these services should be provided at home or in a nursing home cannot be decided on the basis of assessment tools. You can get a DMS-1 score of 180 and still be cared for at home. If you are responsible what do you want to know about a potential client? If providing care is costing $250.00 a day and all you are getting is $80.00 a day for a client, you are going to do something. What do you need to know? There is no difficulty in trying to develop a good instrument. There have been enough studies done to develop assessment tools. A decision has to be made that everybody has to use it, whether it is a hospital discharge planner starting that process at that end or someone who is assessing a patient who has been identified in the community. As may be seen above, no two demonstrations described are assessing clients in the same way. And there is a problem about potential clients who are paying privately and who often absorb the nursing home debts. Will the same assessments be used for the private pay patients and will they be able to be screened out of homes if they want to go into them? That is not the case today.

Summary

Below is a summary of the key points made about organization of the long-term care system.

(1) *Assessment-referral-gatekeeping by a physically responsible agent.* A uniform procedure is needed to decide where a client is going to go and what are the best services for him in terms of appropriateness, quality of care, and fiscal viability. One of the main responsibilities that the person performing this assessment-gatekeeping function would have is fiscal responsibility. A budget would be given to him and within that budget he would have to determine where clients are to go. In other words, there would be only x amount of money to go around for each x number of people.

(2) *Caseloads.* Small caseloads should be given to each case manager. Five thousand people should comprise the maximum caseload. These caseload limits should be uniform throughout the state with some kind of local authority assuming responsibility for each.

This number of 5,000 is arbitrary: it is the size you would not want to exceed before things start to get too difficult.

(3) *Local authority with fiscal responsibility.* The responsible party should be required to have some of its own financing on the line. Thus, it avoids the pitfall of knowing that one can keep going back to the government for more money which prevents the responsible party from ever having to make tough fiscal decisions.

(4) *Start-up funds.* To be approved as the responsible body a local group should be able to come up with some start-up funds, and those start-up funds should be on the line. In other words, it should be known at the outset that if they run out, the government will not readily supply more and another agency would be designated to take their place. Thus, the local agency would have to make the tough decisions to see that clients receive the most cost-effective and the least costly services.

(5) *The best local agency to play this role.* In all likelihood a wide variety of different groups could be involved, e.g., an arm of the government, a provider, a new group that forms, or a day care center. Minimum standards should be set by the state. Fiscal responsibility could be included among those standards. It should not matter what type of provider agency assumes such responsibility as long as there are not 50 different programs in the state all doing things differently. How to prevent this? Let us consider the school district model. A school district is required to give a minimum number of services, that is, a minimum requirement is set by the state. But, as is well known, this model has its limitations because each district puts in different amounts of money and sometimes offers a very different type of educational package. Thus, in the more affluent communities there is always enough money to deliver many educational services but in poor neighborhoods there is little in the way of resources. Thus far, it is difficult to find a solution for this problem. Consequently, it may not be a good model for long-term care.

Private businesses may develop an interest in this area. Benefits constitute a major cost assumed by business these days and as these costs grow, corporations may decide that they want to have a major say in how health care is distributed to their employees. It is not clear who should bear the major responsibility for long-term care services but it seems clear that nursing homes cannot continue to use up the vast percentage of long-term care resources with no controls. Probably the state cannot afford to build many more nursing home beds because once the nursing home is built, it generates huge costs for many years. Therefore, however long-term care is organized and financed, the emphasis will have to be on community-based, long-term care systems.

Case Management: State of the Art

Goldie Green

INTRODUCTION

This chapter deals with five important factors in determining effective case management. They are:

1. adequacy of coverage for the target population,
2. accessibility of service in terms of location of service—whether it is a single or multi-entry point type of service,
3. length of time required for turning on the service or services being coordinated through the case management system,
4. the possible establishment of equitability or equal criteria for all participants, clients, or patients so that everyone has equal access to service,
5. cost effectiveness (this issue will also be addressed in the next article).

CASE MANAGEMENT: A SHORT BACKGROUND STATEMENT

Case management may be known by many names. Often the names are synonymous with terms associated with social work services, such as central registry; protective services; central intake; integrated services; comprehensive casework; client tracking; client monitoring; community-based, long-term care—and the list goes on.

Goldie Green is Research Consultant, Brookdale Institute on Aging and Adult Human Development, Columbia University, New York, N.Y.

This paper was presented along with the participation of the following panel members: Vicki Ashton, Bill Gould, and Rochelle Lipkowitz.

According to one author (Carter, 1978), case management is essentially a recycling of tested concepts going back to the turn of the century. Carter traces the coordination function of case management services to the settlement house and community center focus on the family. Services (child care, nutrition education, legal counseling about immigration laws, recreation) were intended to assist the immigrant families in becoming a part of the American life stream. Social Service Exchanges, which gained momentum in the early 1900s, were also intended in theory to enhance service coordination. In actual practice, however, the exchanges were concerned with preventing duplication of relief-giving. Efforts at coordination during the mid-century (late '40s, early '50s) included the St. Paul Multi-Problem Family Experiment which attempted to facilitate planning and service coordination for those families using a disproportionate share of the service. As with the Social Service Exchanges, a major objective of the service was to conserve scarce resources; however, the St. Paul program was equally concerned with more effective rehabilitation of the families being served.

Subsequent to World War II the concept of "access" was applied (although not necessarily identified as such) to information services for returning veterans eligible for service-connected benefits. The program was considered highly successful; nevertheless, Congress stopped funding it, and the program was phased out by 1949. Continuum of care, another concept associated with case management, emerged in the literature of the '50s. Discovery of medications for psychiatric disorders permitted wide-scale discharges from mental hospitals. Continuum of care referred to ongoing services for patients discharged to the community.

The foregoing have all been concepts associated with case management as well as social work. How then does case management differ from other programs? To begin with, the term case management began to appear in the literature in the early '70s. A watershed in public welfare was reached in mid-1971 with the legislation to separate income maintenance from social services. Shortly before that time, efforts had been directed toward applying "systems theory" to delivery of services and by 1971 the literature abounded with models. An American Public Welfare Association model, for instance, required that the agency maintain a "service inventory" of tangible, specific services—for example, transportation, housing, health care—to assure delivery on user demand. Entry into the system was through a "programmer" who directed the user to the requested service. Services were supplied either (1) from within the agency itself; (2) through (contract) purchase from outside agencies; and/or (3) by "compact," that is, obtained from an outside agency without cost. Around the same time a model was introduced at the National Conference on Social Welfare. The spokesperson (Pauley, 1971) defined the goal of redesigning a community social service system as pulling social service activities together at the delivery level in a manner that would assure accessibility, availability, and responsiveness to the needs and desires of the people served.

Other similar models emerged: Rosenberg and Brody (1974) in *Systems Serving People* cite four, one of which mentions a case manager. Irrespective of the title, that is, whether it is programmer, service manager, or case manager, the actor is identified as being at the hub of the service delivery system. The job description is to assess client needs and then route the client accordingly, to internal and external service providers. All requests for services not agreed upon in the initial service plan were to be channeled through the service manager for rescheduling. Monitoring of services is presented in the model as an integral part of the design. The service manager (or case manager) is to receive feedback from in-house service specialists, consumers, and/or external providers. Evaluation of one of the first APWA models revealed that (1) users did not request all of the services they needed and (2) little effort was extended to coordinate services outside the agency, particularly voluntary services. Rosenberg and Brody, in the four models they explored, found that access to services was greatly improved but, as was reported in the APWA evaluation study, coordination of services from outside resources was less developed than integration of services within the agency.

In brief, case managers "programmed" services to be supplied either from within the agency, through purchase of service, or from sources outside the agency provided without cost. The intent was to assure accessibility, availability, and responsiveness to the needs and desires of the people being served.

Case Management in Long-Term Care

The emergence of case management as an integral part of a social service delivery system was briefly described above. Recently, this concept has been applied to long-term care. In the early '70s, at about the time the APWA models were being developed, Robert

Morris (1971), at the Levinson Gerontological Policy Institute of Brandeis, submitted to Congress a recommendation for a personal care organization that would provide in-home services to the frail elderly in need of long-term care. An initial demonstration program in Massachusetts using the Morris model had little success. Institutionalization for the frail elderly was still the prevailing attitude; in-home services were not viewed as acceptable alternatives. By the mid-1970s, however, further refinement of the proposal for in-home services included a case management component and at about the same time several new demonstration programs were begun. The first and most successful was Triage, in Plainville, Connecticut. Others included the Philadelphia Corporation for Aging and AC-CESS, which is described in Part II above. A statewide program was begun in Georgia, and three separate sites were selected in Wisconsin for a program emanating from the office of the Lt. Governor. Although no two programs during that period were alike, each had case management as a core component.

More recently, new demonstration programs have been organized under federal government funding including the channeling grant which is also described in Part II above. The purpose of the channeling grant is to test out policies that are applicable at the local level. The Robert Wood Johnson Foundation grant to Erie County—also described in Part II above—is funded under voluntary auspices. It is intended to test out concepts applicable to setting policies for case management services (for programs for the elderly) at the state level—in this instance for New York State.

Factors to Be Considered in Evaluating Case Management Services

Crucial factors that must be considered are:

1. Adequacy of coverage, that is, who gets served?
2. Accessibility—can the user find the case management service? Are case managers readily available?
3. Equitability—does every eligible person have the same opportunity to receive needed services?
4. Feasibility—can the program work?
5. Cost-efficiency—can dollar comparisons be made for services with as opposed to those without case management, or for institutional as opposed to in-home services?

1. *Adequacy of coverage* refers to determination of target populations. Ideally, the target population selected for each program is based on community need and community resources. Where resources are in short supply a narrow definition of the target population would be expected as, for instance, those at highest risk of institutionalization or those with no other means of obtaining needed services. Some examples of narrow definition of target population are the Wisconsin Community Care Organization programs where risk of institutionalization, the criterion for admission into the case management program, was identified by a standardized screening device, the Geriatric Functional Rating Scale. Issues of reliability and validity were not gone into in any detail in this demonstration. Because of the narrow definition the target population was extremely difficult to locate and not all of the resources, although meager, were fully utilized.

The Philadelphia Corporation on Aging (PCA) is another example of a program with a very narrowly defined target population. The PCA considers itself a provider of last resort and only those persons unable to find services under any other auspices are provided services administered through PCA. A major role is played by the case manager who is expected to first explore with the client all other resources for meeting the client's needs. This includes family and friends as well as health care programs. Clients who are not eligible for other services and who have no other resources may then receive services administered by the PCA. Although this definition of a target population is highly restrictive, under conditions of scarce resources the program provides services to people who might otherwise remain unserved.

SEQCOAS-JSPOA, also described in Part II above, serves the vulnerable elderly, that is, anyone experiencing stress who needs more than one service. The Monroe County Program, ACCESS, described in Part II above, offers case management services to all income groups using as its eligibility criterion the risk of institutionalization. They found that because of funding arrangements they were limited to implementing plans for Medicaid-eligible clients primarily. Case management serves no purpose for clients in the ACCESS model who need services which they cannot afford (usually the near poor).

Programs under the auspices of Area Agencies on Aging, such as those in Portland and throughout Massachusetts, which provide services to clients on a sliding fee scale, undoubtedly run into similar difficulties (as ACCESS) with clients who cannot afford all of the needed services.

Target populations may differ from one case management program to another. A major issue, under adequacy of coverage, is whether or not the program is capable of serving all of the people who are eligible under the program definition of the target population.

2. *Accessibility*, as stated above refers to (a) the location of case management services in the community and (b) the availability of case managers.* Case management may be centralized or decentralized. The intent of case management services is for the client to have a point of entry into the service system. Ideally, the client is assigned a case manager at the outset who arranges for necessary services. Thus the client no longer has to make separate applications to a variety of resources. The structural design of access points (that is, the point at which the user enters the system) differs in the various models. The major dichotomy is a central intake point versus multiple intake points. And the contact may originate with other sources such as a hospital discharge unit or an information and referral service or a meals-on-wheels program, etc.

There are advantages and disadvantages to both the centralized and the decentralized intake models. For example, a centralized intake point generally has only one telephone number which everyone may call; the decentralized intake point allows for entry through a variety of local resources already known within a community. However, whether or not case management services are accessible to a client is contingent on the availability of case managers. Single entry case coordination services employ staff specifically to do case management. Where access to case management services is through service providers in the community, workers may be assigned case management tasks in addition to their other assignments. They may not have the kind of training or experience to meet the demands of the job and/or they may not be given the kinds of supports and supervision necessary to maintain themselves on the job. A high degree of reliability of case management performance in a single en-

---

*Accessibility, as it is used here, refers to client access to case management. Case management, however, is considered an access service, that is, it provides a means of connecting users to needed services. Other kinds of access services include information and referral services, transportation, entitlement counseling, etc.

try system is assured only if the staff is capable of handling the workload on an ongoing basis.

Triage of Connecticut is an example of a centralized intake system. A single telephone number is available for all clients. As a demonstration program Triage served a target number of clients. A great many were wait-listed before gaining entry into the program, and in the demonstration phase, the agency experienced serious back-up problems.*

PCA is an example of a decentralized system. At least one worker in each of the 33 Senior Centers financed through PCA has been designated a case manager. In addition, PCA has multiple routes to a case manager. These include (a) an information and referral hotline, (b) hospital referrals for non-Medicare/Medicaid-reimbursed home services through a uniform procedure, (c) agency referrals from agencies already providing a needed service through a uniform procedure, and (d) direct contact with the Senior Center closest to where the client lives. The most widely used route is the information and referral hotline. PCA case management accessibility, however, is constrained by an uneven response time. Clients are assigned to case managers on a geographic basis, that is, to intake points closest to where they live. Some case managers can respond immediately while others cannot. In a decentralized system, such as PCA's, it is not usually possible to relocate case managers on the basis of user demand for service.

The issue of accessibility, as described above, refers not only to whether clients can easily locate needed case management services, but whether they can be accepted into the system when they need it.

3. *Equitability* refers to all eligible persons having the same opportunity to receive needed services. That is, is need for service established in the same way for all persons who apply for case management services? Equitability is highly dependent on the assessment process.

Assessment is the most technical aspect of the case management/ service coordination process. Assessment tools may be dichotomized into standard vs. judgmental instruments. When a standard instrument is used, an assessment is reached based on quantitatively established norms, and services are offered the client according to

*Triage currently has a new name, Connecticut Community Care, Inc., and enjoys a new status as a statewide, non-profit, partially state-supported corporation. (Note by the editors.)

the level of care indicated by a score. Instruments are regarded as judgmental when a profile of the client is arrived at qualitatively and services are offered on a discretionary basis. In many of the case management/service coordination models a variety of instruments are used to identify the needs of a given client. In addition, specific kinds of clinical examinations conducted by physicians, nurses, occupational therapists, etc. may be included in a comprehensive assessment. Generally, the purpose of the assessment is to determine what combination of services is necessary to stabilize an individualized client.

Most case management models develop their own assessment instruments. A wide range of standard instruments are also in use. For the most part all assessment instruments cover the person's physical, mental, and social needs and include living conditions and functioning status. Explorations with family and other natural supports in the environment (neighbors, friends, etc.) are also a part of a comprehensive assessment.

Of major concern to the issue of equitability of case management is that the same instrument be used for assessment of the entire target population, and that persons doing the assessment have uniform skills and/or professional expertise so that all clients have the same opportunity to receive a needed service. Equitability as applied to assessment instruments includes the notion that neither more nor less service than is needed be offered to a client. The intent of equitability in many case management programs is to insure maximum independence and the least restrictive service package.

Examples of variations in choice of assessment instruments areas follow:

(1) Triage used a battery of tests, some standard, some judgmental. The standard tests that were used were: Activities of Daily Living (Katz et al.); Instrumental Activities of Daily Living (Lawton & Brody); and The Mental Status Questionnaire (Kahn et al.). In addition, a comprehensive form was developed and refined by the project director, the project research team, and the geriatric physician consultant. The assessment forms were intended to cover health and social history including an evaluation of housing, transportation, finances, nutritional status, and other social needs; the patient's/client's physical, mental, and social needs, including present living conditions and functioning status; a modified physical examination performed by a nurse-clinician which included, but was not limited to, hearing and visual measurement, cardio-pulmonary and

musculoskeletal evaluation, and urinalysis. Any symptomatology mentioned by the client during the health history was further evaluated during the physical assessment. The information gathered was then organized and charted using Lawrence Weed's problem-oriented approach.

(2) ACCESS also has a strong assessment component with a capability of prescreening for level of care. Clients may be returned to their homes rather than transferred from one institution to another if the ACCESS assessment indicates home care as a preferable alternative. ACCESS also has the capability of recommending a decision for home care based on the assessment and irrespective of other opinions.

(3) PCA has a simplified assessment instrument that is easy to administer, but it is oriented to screening clients out rather than in (as a provider of last resort).

(4) Portland has no structured assessment. Programs in the Portland area are considered providers of last resort for case management services. In other words, if a client is unable to make the necessary contacts for services and has no family or friends to help, Portland case managers can assist. The client's need for services is established on a discretionary or judgmental basis.

There are a number of sources of complexity: (1) Professional status—whether or not health care services are being coordinated is a factor to be considered, since only a health care professional may authorize such services. Using highly trained professionals, such as nurse/social worker teams, both of whom have master level degrees, may prevent highly discretionary judgments, but it is costly. (2) Time is another complicating factor. Comprehensive assessments are lengthy procedures. Information cannot always be obtained in one interview. Assessments are frequently done in steps over an extended period. Where there is a high demand for service, either the case managers become bogged down with assessments and cannot implement plans, or the clients are kept waiting for service for extended periods.

Some of the programs attempt to get around these complexities. ACCESS case managers authorize completion of specific assessment instruments by respective professionals on an as-needed basis. This includes—in addition to medical, nursing, and psychosocial assessment—finance counseling, home assessment (architectural limitation), and social work assessment of informal support systems (family, friends). PCA arranges for assessments to be done by referral sources where professional expertise is available, thus freeing up case managers to direct their energies to other aspects of the case management service. On the other hand, Triage case managers conducted their own assessments. The time spent doing them was most likely balanced out by the ready availability of services under their purchase-of-service arrangements.

Whether or not a program can provide service equitably may be determined, in large part, by: (1) use of a single assessment instrument for all users of the service, (2) by insuring that all persons doing the assessment have uniform skills and/or professional expertise, and (3) by taking time into consideration in applying assessments.

4. *Feasibility* refers to whether or not a plan can be implemented and monitored. Putting a client through a well-structured intake system is of no value if the services needed are not available. A variety of means have been found to coordinate provider services. Case management/service coordination may start out with direct control of funding sources for purchase of service, or may obtain waivers for control of third party payments. Some programs attempt voluntary agreements with providers. Where no provider coordination exists, case managers negotiate for services from community agencies on a case-by-case basis. For instance, PCA has a program with most assurance of feasibility since it coordinates the services it funds. However, case managers must independently coordinate services not provided through the network.

ACCESS, Triage, and the Wisconsin CCOs all had federal government waivers for purchase of service. The ACCESS waivers allowed for authorization of social services as well as health-related services under Medicaid. As previously mentioned, some clients not eligible for Medicaid could not afford some services they needed. An interesting aside is that though ACCESS could authorize some social services for Medicaid payment, an evaluation study conducted during the third year found that the social services were not used. ACCESS case managers have to "shop" for services since ACCESS does not have a coordinated provider network. Triage waivers permitted purchase of service through contract. Triage developed a coordinated provider network and encouraged development of resources in short supply. However, the Triage demonstration program coordinated only those services under purchase of service contract. Triage case managers would give verbal authorization for a necessary service from an agency under contract to it and would then follow-up with a formal agreement. The Wisconsin-CCO waivers were of limited advantage. Waivers were obtained essentially for health-related services. Other services had to be negotiated by the case manager on a case-by-case basis. An added wrinkle in the Wisconsin CCOs was the maintenance-of-service effort which required that clients continue with services they were already receiving. Thus, the Wisconsin programs had no control over all of the services and the barriers to monitoring quantity and quality were difficult to breach.

As might be surmised from the above, provider coordination is the most difficult job the case manager has to perform. Provider coordination entails obtaining agreements from providers to (1) accept uniform assessment as the basis for complying with a request for service, (2) respect the case manager's monitoring decisions, and (3) accept reassessment decisions for termination of services. Where purchase-of-service contracts exist, the buyer has the prerogative of determining how and when a service will be used. However, where voluntary agreements exist, the provider is being asked to give up control over services for which the provider agency is accountable. On the other hand, the advantages of case management services are lost without some working arrangement with providers. It is highly unlikely that case managers can perform their job effectively if they must negotiate every case with every provider. If a service is requested and improperly implemented, the case manager is in the unpleasant position of having to work out the problem with the provider. Despite a high level of training, experience, and good will, case managers have been reported to "burn out" quickly. Average length of stay on the job ranges from about 6 months to 2 years. This works against the advantages of the case management process, since some case continuity is lost in the change-over of case managers.

A community approach to organizing providers is highly stressful for the staff involved, and there is no guarantee of results. Some provider groups maintain their own autonomy and gain strength from the numbers in their professional associations.

Monitoring and reassessment are both contingent upon provider agreements. Follow-up or monitoring to ensure delivery of agreed-upon services is an integral part of case management. It is a primary role of the case manager, and unless the position carries some authority to perform this function, the case manager has little influence over the process of bringing about a change in the quality or quantity of service being provided. This was a lesson learned from the Wisconsin-CCO demonstrations for which requirement of a maintenance-of-service effort meant that case managers had to develop case plans around the services a client was receiving at the time. As much as we would like to think that all services are provided in the best interest of the client, we know, in fact, that some services may be inadequate and that others may be extraneous. Monitoring and reassessment are expected to be done at regular intervals to determine if any changes are needed in the service plans. Unless the case managers have authority to reauthorize, change, or terminate services, they cannot perform this part of their job. Reassessment may be done by someone other than the case manager such as special evaluation personnel, but the case manager still requires authority for a change in service plan.

Thus, the feasibility of a case management program is primarily dependent upon the availability of needed services. The services may be coordinated in many ways; however, for a program to be feasible the case manager will need to be able to locate efficiently services to implement a case plan. Monitoring the service and reassessment are also important case management functions and are most likely to be carried out effectively when the case manager has the necessary authority to negotiate changes with the providers.

5. *Cost Efficiency.* All case management models have as one of many objectives the efficient use of resources. At first glance, cost efficiency may seem like a simple proposition. One might ask, "Which program provides the most service for the least amount of money?" Answers, however, are not easily found. Some programs, for instance, have attempted to compare unit costs of service provided through case management programs with unit costs of services obtained by clients in control groups that have not received case management services. However, these models can only measure cost effectiveness (which program costs less) when the programs have the same objectives. Comparison of the cost of maintaining a person at home with the cost of institutionalization, per person, have met with similar difficulties. For instance, one elderly person may be receiving in-home services because family members are available to assist while another elderly person may be institutionalized because no family or friends are available. Case management may give an elderly person the choice of remaining at home

whether or not family or friends are available to assist, but the cost of in-home services may exceed the cost of institutional services. Though where quality issues are compared, the balance might shift in favor of in-home services. Needless to say, all the data are not in and the cost efficiency of case management programs remains an open issue.

Summary and Conclusions

Case management services have been used in many ways not touched upon in the foregoing material. This presentation was essentially focused on case management as a major component of an in-home service delivery system for the elderly. It was noted that many concepts of case management—service coordination, access, continuum of care—had been applied in other contexts in the past. The uniqueness of case management as part of a long-term care service delivery system was noted. Five factors relevant to case management programs were discussed. They are: (1) adequacy of coverage, (2) accessibility, (3) equitability, (4) feasibility, and (5) cost efficiency. Advantages and disadvantages relevant to these five factors were described for selected programs. No one program seemed to have all of the advantages. Critical appraisal of case management programs is needed to help determine more effective ways of delivering services.

A number of important and as yet unsolved issues involved in case management remain to be considered: (1) How do you target the population? For example, do you target on the basis of types of services they need, the number of services they need, or their age? (2) What is an assessment? What is it actually looking for? What is a comprehensive assessment? What do you do after you have an assessment? (3) How do you do case management when needed services are not in place or when the services are so scarce that you have to put a patient on a waiting list? And how do you manage a case when there are no services? (4) What happens to the persons being managed? (5) What is involved in interagency service coordination?

One thing is clear and that is that coordination is essential. If there is not a provider coordination network of some sort or communication between providers, then the rest of the system that is put into place will not work. It probably is crucial for cost effectiveness. There are those who think that if you look at all the individual systems added up, a case management system may not necessarily be cheaper. In some cases it may even be more expensive. But that gets one into the issue of quality of care. Is the quality of what is being provided better? There seems to be no resolution of this perpetually raised dilemma.

The underlying philosophy of case management should be comprehensive care. The entry point into the system may come from medical, mental health, or social service agencies. The care provider may be a nurse, doctor, social worker, or paraprofessional. Within the social agency, the manager's discipline may not be as important as his/her commitment to providing the best possible care for the individual.

Case management may have to be conducted very sensitively. One must guard against creating dependency in either individuals or agencies. This requires a determination of how much the natural support system is doing, how much the provider network is doing, and how much the public systems are doing. Ultimately, who is responsible for making decisions? Is it the case manager, the client, the natural support system, or the reimbursement mechanism that makes decisions about what types of services are turned on and where and when? It was suggested that the case management system had to achieve a balance whereby the family or natural support system had a maximum role in the case management decision making because the family would gain greater satisfaction in getting what they thought they needed and because the family's greater involvement would have cost implications. It was suggested that the more involved the family, the less costly the plan was going to be.

Who will train case managers and in which discipline will this training be lodged is another important issue.

There was a study conducted at Brandeis University which looked at case planning decisions done by physicians, nurses, social workers, and family members. It should not be surprising that every discipline had a different view. Even the family had a different perception. In the instance of families, they all had the perception of need—that what a person needed was to be sustained in the home which meant that home care was what was needed. There were major differences of opinion: obviously the physician wanted more medical visits, the nurse wanted more nursing visits and rehabilitation, the social worker wanted to social work the client to death, and the family wanted personal care and really did not address the medical issues. The moral of this story is that there are major differences in styles of decision making depending on discipline. Should there be a new discipline of case management? Should graduate schools train case managers?

Case management may be an interdisciplinary discipline like planning. There are different specialties within planning, e.g., city planning, health planning, etc. But planning is a generic discipline with specialized skills and a knowledge base. Perhaps case management could follow a similar route. For case management to be effective the following conditions probably should prevail: (1) The community has to have a fairly integrated service delivery system network in place. (2) There have to be adequate support services that can be called upon outside of those immediately made available by the participating agencies. (3) The essence of coordination is communication. If agencies are not part of a communication network, whatever management system you set up will not work.

Case management is a tool for turning on and providing services; it is not a panacea. It will not solve problems if the network itself is made up of agencies who are not willing to be honest with one another and to share information with one another.

BIBLIOGRAPHY

Alternatives to Nursing Home Care: A Proposal. Prepared for Use by the Special Committee on Aging, United States Senate, by Staff Specialists at the Levinson Gerontological Institute, Brandeis University, Waltham, MA. October 1971.

Carter, Genevieve. "Service Coordination: A Recycling of Tested Concepts." National Conference on Social Welfare, Los Angeles, May 1978. (Distributed by the Social Policy Laboratory, Ethel Percy Andrus Gerontology Center, University of Southern California.)

City of Portland. Oregon Human Resource Bureau, Contract Package on Case Management.

Gottesman, Leonard E., Ishizaki, Barbara, and MacBride, Stacey Mong. "Service Management—Plan and Concept in Pennsylvania." *The Gerontologist*, 1979, *19*(4), 379-385.

Hicks, Barbara C. Principal Research Investigator. Triage: Coordinated Delivery of Services to the Elderly. Final Report, Connecticut State Department on Aging, December 1979.

Ishizaki, Barbara, Gottesman, Leonard E., and MacBride, Stacey Mong. "Determinants of Model Choice for Service Management Systems." *The Gerontologist*, 1979, *19*(4), 385-388.

Kahn, Alfred J. "Public Social Services: The Next Phase—Policy and Delivery Strategies." *Public Welfare*, Winter 1972, 15-24.

Long-Term Care for the 1980's: Channeling Demonstrations and Other Initiatives. Hearings Before the Subcommittee on Health and Long-Term Care of the Select Committee on Aging, House of Representatives, Ninety-Sixth Congress, Second Session, February 27, 1980.

Macro Systems, Inc. Third Year Evaluation of the Monroe County Long-Term Care Program, 1980. Prepared for New York State Department of Social Services and the Health Care Financing Administration by Lewis C. Price, Hinda M. Ripps, David M. Piltz.

The Massachusetts Department of Elder Affairs. Boston, MA, Home Care, Area Agencies on Aging.

Morris, Robert and Anderson, Delwin. "Personal Care Services: An Identity for Social Work." *Social Service Review*, June 1975, *49*, 157-174.

Pauley, Ruth M. Redesigning a Social Service Delivery System, Social Work Practice, National Conference on Social Welfare. New York: Columbia University Press, 1971, 139-151.

Philadelphia Corporation for Aging. Area Plan for Aging, Summary and Supplement, 1981-1983.

Quinn, Joan L. and Rieck, David W. "Triage—An Alternative Approach to Care of the Elderly." National Journal's Conference "The Economics of Aging," November 30-December 1, 1978, Washington, D.C.

Rosenberg, Marvin and Brody, Ralph. Systems Serving People: A Breakthrough in Service Delivery. Case Western Reserve University, School of Applied Social Sciences. Cleveland, Ohio, 1974.

Schneider, Don. Patient/Client Assessment in New York State, Volumes I and II, May 1980. (Study performed under contract to Schneider and Associates from the Health Planning Commission of New York State.)

Seidl, Fredrick W., Applebaum, Robert, Austin, Carol D., and Mahoney, Kevin J. Delivering In-Home Services to the Aged and Disabled: The Wisconsin Community Care Organization Final Evaluation Report, April 1980.

Steinberg, Raymond. "Case Coordination: Lessons from the Past for Future Program Models." National Conference on Social Welfare, Los Angeles, May 1978. (Distributed by the Social Policy Laboratory, Ethel Percy Andrus Gerontology Center, University of Southern California.)

Weed, Lawrence L. Medical Records, Medical Education and Patient Care. Cleveland, Ohio: The Press of Case Western Reserve University, 1971.

Case Management:
A Service Package

Vicki Ashton, MSW

Introduction

The following paper provides a description of an AoA funded demonstration project that was carried out through the Southeast Queens Consortium of Aging Services - SEQCOAS (as described in Part II). Case management is defined as a service package designed to bring resources to those who cannot coordinate resources on their own. The project attempted to test two models of case management: one was computer supported and one used the team approach.

Project Description

Case management, an old concept with new applications, is being tested in various settings as a way of stretching limited resources to reach a growing clientele. One such effort is the Southeast Queens Consortium of Aging Services (SEQCOAS). SEQCOAS is a three-year demonstration project funded by AoA and developed and administered by the Jamaica Service Program for Older Adults (JSPOA), a multi-service agency for the elderly in Queens, New York. SEQCOAS has three major components:

1. A formal consortium of 32 agencies providing service to the elderly in Southeast Queens.
2. A computer system designed to be used by individual consortium members according to their capabilities, while still producing information of value to the entire consortium.
3. A voluntary, interagency case management system supported by the computerized Management Information System.

Vicki Ashton is Consultant, Columbia University Center for Geriatrics and Gerontology, New York, N.Y.

The SEQCOAS case management model can be viewed as a logical end step in a coordinated service system. SEQCOAS members recognized that each agency in the consortium has its own internal method of case management. Consequently, the system developed does not supplant individual agency effort, but is a way of helping frail clients through various levels of intervention, often among several providers.

SEQCOAS estimates that 19% of the total 70,000 aged population in Southeast Queens is frail or vulnerable. The two terms are used interchangeably to refer to persons who, because of one or more physical, mental, or social impairment, cannot obtain needed services. Many frail elderly are relatively isolated and unaware of services beyond entitlements such as Social Security and Medicare. Those who are aware are discouraged from seeking help by complicated, often physically exhausting application procedures. The problem is worse when more than one service is needed.

Case management addresses the needs of the frail elderly as a group and individualizes service for each person within the group. SEQCOAS case management can be defined as a service package designed to bring resources to those who cannot coordinate resources on their own. The ultimate goal of the project is to make service delivery accessible, comprehensive, integrated, and accountable to this population.

In developing the project, SEQCOAS addressed the following issues:

- Evaluation of concepts for interagency case management
- Development of interagency agreements for case management responsibility
- Development of common assessment and service plan forms
- Development of common definitions and units of service
- Definition of the target population for case management services including a definition of vulnerability
- Establishment of procedures to protect client confidentiality

In October 1980, SEQCOAS received a supplemental AoA grant to support the development of the case management project, with the following aims:

1. To test two models of voluntary, interagency case management directed toward the frail elderly. Model I is computer supported; Model II is a team approach.

2. To identify and eliminate gaps in the current system of services to the frail and vulnerable and to determine how the service system can be made more effective and efficient in meeting the needs of this population.

3. To improve communication between SEQCOAS and the federal and state funding agencies to permit localities to contribute in developing national service priorities and enable funding agencies to benefit from and respond to innovative approaches to service provision at the local level.

Once the grant was received, SEQCOAS notified member agencies and encouraged participation. Start up required more time and effort than anticipated due to various staff levels involved. Member agency administrative staff agreed to participate in the project and assigned line staff as case managers. This required two sets of orientation and training, one so that administrative staff could sanction the service and incorporate it within their agencies; the other so that line staff could relate the service to everyday realities of client needs and worker capabilities, particularly since staff assumed case management duties in addition to their regular assignments.

Flexibility was crucial to the development of the project. When many different agencies are involved, each with its own direct service agenda, there is no one set of ground rules that will suit all. SEQCOAS met this challenge by permitting units of agencies to participate instead of the entire agency. Flexibility was also needed regarding eligibility criteria. When the project started, the major criterion for client selection was that the person be frail and require services from more than one provider. However, an interesting trend became apparent. Except for federal entitlement programs, social service agencies had moved away from single service delivery toward diversification. In Southeast Queens, senior centers, which, a few years ago, offered only lunch, have expanded into multi-purpose centers providing a range of programs and services to the aged, from entitlement advocacy to home care. Consequently, once an elderly person enters the service system, many available services can be provided at the point of entry. SEQCOAS changed client selection criteria to reflect the environment: To be eligible for case management service, a frail older person must require assistance in coordinating more than one resource, inter- or intra-agency.

Nine agencies, including JSPOA, participate; 4 in the computer model and 5 in the team approach. JSPOA participates in both. The project is directed by a case management coordinator, responsible to the SEQCOAS director. Each model, as far as possible given the small numbers, includes a mix of health and social service agencies. There are written agreements between SEQCOAS and agencies participating in Model I outlining the terms of computer utilization. A computer terminal is stationed at each agency participating in Model I.

Participating agencies designate a staff person from an appropriate unit or section to serve as case manager in the selected model. Non-participating agencies designate a staff person to act as liaison to both computer and team models to facilitate referrals and follow through.

For the project, agency case managers use SEQCOAS data collection forms. Participating staff received initial orientation from the case management coordinator on the parameters, procedures, and goals of the project. Ongoing training focuses on resource development, entitlement updates, and service coordination at the client level.

Model I: Computer Supported

In this model the case manager works individually and uses the computer directly at each phase of the process. At intake, if the client meets the criteria for case management, the computer is used to determine if the person is known to one of the other eight agencies participating in the project. Assessment and service plan information is fed into the computer. Service is arranged as needed. Referrals to other agencies are made directly through other case managers or appointed liaisons. If the second agency is part of the computer-assisted model, only the client identification number is needed by the receiving case manager who can then obtain demographic, assessment, service plan, and service delivery information directly from the computer. This type of computer utilization protects the older person from unnecessary duplication and saves time for case managers. Summarized information can be reviewed at a glance and changes and additions can be made promptly.

Model II: Team Approach

In the team approach, the computer is used for all phases of case management, however, the team, not the individual, acts as the case manager. The individual manager does an intake and assessment at the point of entry and submits the material to the case management coordinator who reviews the information, puts it into the central computer, and schedules a team meeting to discuss the case. The team, with the client's participation, makes a service plan and maintains responsibility for its implementation and follow-up. For the older person's convenience, one agency representative is designated as the client's primary contact.

The team meets whenever there is a new case to be presented, a problem on an existing case, or a reassessment. The case manager presents information to the group, and the computer printouts are used to enrich the discussion. Since most case management cases need an array of services, the general SEQCOAS membership is used as a resource pool and representatives are invited to team meetings as needed to provide assistance on relevant cases. Project operations revealed other issues:

- Case management is not appropriate for all frail elderly. Older people who are very impaired and or caught up with living and dying may not even be approachable. This often occurs in a hospital setting.
- The agency setting may preclude the practicality of case management. Hospital in-patient units do not carry patients long enough to warrant setting up case management within that unit.
- The SEQCOAS project is easily affected by changes within participating agencies. For example, one of the mental health agencies had a geriatric unit which participated in the case management project. The entire agency underwent a reorganization based on geographic categories rather than age. The geriatric unit was disbanded and an outpatient clinic was substituted which had a large elderly population within their locale.
- The turfdom issue remains. Each agency feels it can provide the most appropriate case management service for its clients.

Despite these problems the case management project provides a model of how service integration at the systems level can be successfully translated to improved service delivery at the client level. Both models of SEQCOAS interagency case management center on the needs and strengths of the older person. The older person is seen as the person most knowledgeable about his situation and is expected and encouraged to participate in the full process as much as possible. For the very old or frail person, the idea of working with service providers is alien. SEQCOAS case management facilitates client participation by building on the person's strengths in order to foster independence and self-worth.

Both models involve six phases or steps: assessment, development of a service plan, implementation of the plan, follow-up and monitoring, reassessment, and termination.

Assessment

The SEQCOAS assessment form is an eight-page form designed to look at the older person's daily functioning and social networks.

A comprehensive assessment is the foundation of case management. An assessment highlights the important features of a person's life, identifies current needs and problems, and indicates potential areas of stress. The assessment and the service plan are interrelated. Services and resources can be identified and scheduled in a systematic way. The client does not have to wait for a crisis to receive attention. A proper assessment can reduce anxiety by prioritizing needs and scheduling service delivery. For an isolated older person, with decreasing capabilities, it can be a great relief to know that meals will be delivered or arrangements made for congregate meals if and when necessary.

A major part of the SEQCOAS case manager's role in making an assessment and service plan is to help the client and the client's family identify those areas where the older person can manage independently, areas where the person can benefit from help from natural supports, and areas where the case manager will provide major assistance. The SEQCOAS assessment form categorizes natural supports by accessibility, i.e., persons who are available within 30 minutes, beyond 30 minutes, and persons who are not readily available but are significant in the client's life. This type of specific information helps the client and worker determine how to utilize assistance from family, friends, and neighbors.

Service Plan, Development, and Implementation

The service plan depends on the older person's needs and the availability of resources. The SEQCOAS experience indicates that direct service must be readily available in order for case management to work. SEQCOAS found that within the target community home care services are in particularly short supply. Virtually all home care providers have waiting lists, some longer than others. At times the case manager can develop a service plan adjusted to provider waiting lists and schedules, while helping the client cope until service arrives. However, where there are glaring deficiencies between need and resources, case management cannot work.

Interagency communication and cooperation facilitate development and implementation of the service plan. Both the SEQCOAS computer-supported and team approach benefit from strong interagency ties and coordination. The team model actively utilizes interagency relationships. The assessment, which is done at point of entry, is reviewed by the team along with the client and available family or interested persons. Through collective effort, the team delineates the responsibility of each agency, maximizes resources, and develops workable alternatives if parts of the service plan cannot be implemented.

Follow-Up and Monitoring

Categorical programs are set up so that it is possible for half a dozen service providers, or units of one provider, to be in direct contact with a client. Differences in scheduling and personalities can be overwhelming. The SEQCOAS case manager acts as a buffer between the frail older person and the service system, permitting the client to manage those parts he or she feels capable of handling. By working together, the client and the worker set up schedules and determine the appropriateness of the services delivered.

Reassessment

Reassessment serves two purposes. It permits a continued exploration of the older person's life-style and coping patterns, and it measures progress toward the goals set out in the service plan. SEQ-COAS experience indicates that reassessment for the frail elderly should be done 30 to 60 days after the initial assessment.

Termination

Much of the literature on case management recommends termination of case management services once needed services are in place. However, SEQCOAS has found that for the frail elderly, case management consists of more than bringing a one time service to the client. Case management services for the frail elderly may need to be sustained for the duration of the client's life and must be adaptable to the person's needs. Case managers working with the elderly must be aware that the older person's ability to manage any given life event may change over time with dependency increasing and decreasing. Therefore the process of case management can vary from intense, frequent interaction during periods of need and dependency to periods of infrequent contact during times of well-being and relative independence. The case manager must also be aware that very elderly, impaired persons may not progress and that the goal in these situations is one of maintaining the person's present level of functioning.

SEQCOAS' Models: Implications for Practice

Comprehensive, ongoing case management has implications for workers as well as benefits for frail elderly clients. The SEQCOAS model suggests that case management and direct service delivery can co-exist without loss of quality in either service. In addition, by exploring two approaches to case management, SEQCOAS has been able to test the usefulness of each model as it pertains to client and worker needs. Each approach is suitable for particular situations. The computer-assisted model is appropriate for uncomplicated cases where the worker is able to coordinate and monitor services with available supervision and support within the agency. The computer gives the added dimension of information storage and immediate input and retrieval.

The team approach is successful in handling difficult multiproblem situations. The team offers the case manager peer review and support in addition to whatever supervision is available within the worker's agency. Interagency team case management builds on the collective experience of colleagues with different vantage points and skills. The team provides the opportunity for workers to ventilate frustrations, identify underutilized resources, and explore options.

For an ideal case management situation, both computer-assisted and team management should be available to the worker to utilize according to the demands of the case situation and the worker's needs.

Client Characteristics

Thirty-two older persons are being served by the case management project at this time. Data extracted from computer printouts presents a profile of case management clients compared to persons served under title IIIB.* The demographic summary indicates that the case management population is older and poorer than the general population and most in need of home care and transportation services.

	Case Management Clients (%)	Title IIIB Recipients (%)
Age		
80-85+	47	28
Income		
$3,099.00 or Less	21	14
$3,500.00-$3,999.00	30	18
$4,000.00-$4,999.00	8	10
$4,500.00-$4,999.00	21	8
Household Composition		
Live Alone	52	53
With spouse	13	22
With children	21	10
With non-relative	13	5
Functional Limitations		
None	21	33
Walking	65	38
Homebound	65	41
Services Requested		
Entitlements	34	22
Home Care	73	32
Transportation	39	12

*Title IIIB, State funds channelled through the New York City Department for the Aging, provides for a range of services including information, counseling, transportation, housekeeper, and homemaker services.

In an attempt to evaluate what impact case management has on the target group, a case record review was made of five clients in the project and five similar clients (i.e., frail, multi-problem) not in the project. The following observations are the result of that review.

Non-Case Management

1. Information about problems and resources is gathered piece-meal, as the client's service request is seen as an isolated need rather than in relation to all his needs.
2. Client contact with worker is usually around a crisis situation.
3. Both groups of clients have natural supports, e.g., family or neighbors. However, the supports of the non-case management clients were frustrated in their attempts to help the older person and were frequently in need of help themselves.
4. Non-case management clients became confused about various entitlements and the steps needed to obtain them. Consequently they had long delays between the time the need was presented and the service was received.
5. When clients refuse service they get nothing.

Case Management

1. A systematic assessment helps worker and older person identify problems and resources. One service need is viewed in relation to the whole.
2. Systematic assessment and a service plan developed with the client facilitates scheduling service delivery and arranging for alternatives if something goes wrong. Case management prevents breakdowns before they happen.
3. The benefits of case management spread to the client's natural supports. A large part of case management has to do with minimizing stress and helping and supporting the efforts of relatives and friends in assisting their elderly.
4. The case manager works with the client at each step and advocates for the older person as necessary. Services are delivered rapidly, in some cases, immediately.
5. When clients refuse service, which happens most often with Medicaid, alternate care plans are arranged which are more acceptable to the older person.

Although the sample is very small, it is clear that case management can have a positive impact on an older person's life. Problem situations are resolved quickly, and the person is stabilized within a short time.

In the sample, the frail elderly who were not in the project were known to various social service organizations for months, in some cases for more than a year, yet their situations continued to worsen. The non-case-managed clients were generally clients of small senior centers or clubs with limited staff to handle involved, time-consuming problems. Consequently, the clients bounced from one service or entitlement worker to another, becoming more confused in the process. Follow-up was done only when the client came back to the original worker presenting either the same need or a crisis.

As a result of this review, case management services will be offered to those persons not in the project. In addition, ongoing review will be done on active cases within SEQCOAS member agencies to identify potential case management clients.

BIBLIOGRAPHY

Carter, Genevieve, Downing, Rachel, Hutson, Diane, O. and Ishizaki, Barbara S. *Case Coordination with the Elderly: The Experiences of Front-Line Practitioners.* Proceedings and Summary of Findings from the Symposium held January 20-22, 1979, Andrus Gerontology Center. Administration on Aging Grant #90-A-1280.
Case Management: State of the Art. Final Report. Grant No. 54-P-71542/3/-01. Submitted to the Administration on Developmental Disabilities, U.S. Department of Health and Human Services. April 15, 1981.
Coordinating Human Services at the Local Level. Proceedings of the First National Network Building Conference, Denver, Colorado, June 23-24, 1980. Published by Office of Human Development Services, Health and Human Services.
DeWitt, John. "Managing the Human Service System." *Human Service Monograph Series,* August 1977, No. 4.
Gottesman, Leonard and Ishizaki, Barbara. "Service Management-Plan and Concept in Pennsylvania." *The Gerontologist,* 1979. *19*(4), 379-385.
Horton, Gerald T., Carr, Victoria, M.E., and Corcoran, George J. "Illustrating Services Integration from Categorical Bases." *Human Services Monograph Series.* Project Share, November 1976, No. 3.
Ishizaki, Barbara, Gottesman, Leonard, McBride, Stacey Mong. "Determinants of Model Choice for Service Management Systems." *The Gerontologist,* 1979, *19*(4), 385-388.
Jacobs, Bella. *Senior Centers and the At-Risk Older Person.* Washington, D.C.: National Institute of Senior Centers, The National Council on the Aging, 1980, 230.
Taylor, James B. and Gibbons, Jacque. "Microcomputer Applications in Human Service Agencies." *Human Services Monograph Series.* Project Share, November 1980, No. 16.

Costs and Benefits of Expanding In-Home and Community-Based, Long-Term Care Services

Dennis L. Kodner

Introduction

The workshop on costs and benefits raised several important issues and problems concerning the adequacy of research results for public policy development, cost-controlling mechanisms, eligibility criteria, and comparisons of community-based services with institutional care.

The workshop was divided into two parts: one part was devoted to a presentation of the "state of the art" and the other section dealt with a discussion of the main issues.

Summary of the "State of the Art"

The discussion on the "state of the art" included a review of research findings on the impact of expanded in-home and community-based, long-term care services on the following areas: per diem and total costs and outcomes and benefits.

According to the research literature summarized in *Long Term Care: Background and Future Directions*, the U.S. Dept. of Health and Human Services, HCFA-20047, January 1981, the following facts are apparent regarding impacts, per diem, and total costs:

1. A significant number of patients/clients in need of long-term care can be cared for in community settings at lower costs than in institutions.

At the time of this presentation, Mr. Kodner was Director of Planning and Community Services at Metropolitan Jewish Geriatric Center, Brooklyn, N.Y. Elderplan, Inc. is the subsidiary of MJGC responsible for the S/HMO project. This paper was presented along with the participation of Msgr. John J. Barry, cochairman of the workshop.

2. As the individual's level of impairment increases, a "break-even" point is reached whereby nursing home care becomes more economical.
3. Most research on the cost of community care focuses on its impact on public outlays, rather than on total public and private costs (including the imputed costs of informal care).
4. There is little convincing evidence that coverage of community-based and in-home, long-term care services would reduce total public expenditures in an open-ended, fee-for-service system. This is apparently so because these expanded benefits would most likely go to a new or additional service population (the so-called "add-on" population), rather than directly substituting for those who are actually at-risk for nursing home care.

With regard to *outcomes* and *benefits* associated with community long-term care, research findings support the following conclusions:

1. Most long-term care demonstrations report improved contentment and life satisfaction among members of the experimental group.
2. Expanded non-institutional services tend to reduce experimental group mortality.
3. There does not appear to be significant improvement in client functional ability.

Discussion of the Main Issues

1. Is existing research regarding the costs and effects of alternate long-term care programs (e.g., adult day care, home care, etc.) adequate to develop public policy and plan needed services?

The overall consensus of the workshop members was that analysis of existing research on the costs and benefits of community-based and in-home, long-term care services has been motivated from a biased, fixed point of view, i.e., anti-community care, and the research itself, in many instances, was poorly defined and methodologically weak. Key questions such as the impact of these expanded services on total costs (including the costs of hospitalization) as well as the effect of case management on cost control have been almost totally avoided. Therefore, existing research on the costs and benefits of alternate long-term care programs is not entirely adequate for developing policy needed to plan services now and in the future. (The issue of evaluation research is addressed in the next chapter.) However, community care proponents feel strongly that there is enough "real-world" experience to restructure the long-term care system. It is argued that an organized system is better than a fragmented one and that in-home care in most cases is preferable to institutionalization.

In emphasizing home care over nursing home care, one must recognize that there are often two to three times as many people in the community outside of the institution who are at-risk for institutionalization and who may utilize community services (but not nursing homes), thereby upping total long-term care costs. Therefore, there is good reason to move cautiously in making plans to develop a case management system. Needless to say such a system must have cost controls and clearly focus on those individuals at imminent risk of nursing home placement.

2. *Is in-home and community-based, long-term care less costly and more beneficial than nursing home care?*

Workshop participants expressed the "gut" feeling that such services are both less costly and more beneficial. While research findings conclude that community care has a positive impact on "quality of life" (see previous reference HCFA, 1981), participants admitted great difficulty in finding "proof" for the cost savings point of view. Part of the problem in answering this question is the variability of older peoples' needs and the fact that we do not know enough about long-term care intervention strategies to determine what approaches work and which are most cost effective.

Institutional care is often provided when community care of one sort or another does not work. Some people reach a point where the informal support system breaks down or the level of disability gets to be so great that the individual can no longer be safely and comfortably maintained in the community. We are, of course, referring to a highly individualized "breaking point." We do not know where that point is for any given caregiver. Thus, it is hard to compare institutionalized with non-institutionalized people if they are not comparable in this sense. As a result, research cannot clearly answer the question of whether or not nursing homes are more or less effective than community-based services.

Data from most HCFA-supported demonstrations show reduced per diem costs for program clients, but raise the issue that a great

number of these individuals would never have been institutionalized. What this implies is that expanded home care would increase
the nation's long-term care bill. The basic research design needed to
answer this question would consist of comparing two people with
the same score on a DMS-1 form or another comprehensive assessment instrument and assign one to a community care and the other to
nursing home care; preferably the two should be "twins." Research
results should show that one person does quite well after a given
period of time while the other does not. Costs would also be computed to measure cost benefit. Thus far, no research has produced
such clear-cut results.

3. *Do expanded non-institutional services supplant rather than
supplement informal caregiving? What are the cost implications?*

Workshop members recognized the potential for non-institutional
care to supplant family caregiving, thus greatly driving up the costs
of long-term care services.

Community-based services are certainly not more cost effective if
they replace informal family supports. This issue is important for
future policy. It may well be the case that the nature of the family is
changing and that the level of support is probably going to dwindle.
Family support, needless to say, is rather important from a public
point of view because it costs the public sector nothing or very little.
But, we are unsure about whether the expansion of community-
based services will supplement the informal caregiving network or
supplant it.

Existing long-term care experiments did not demonstrate that
such substitution has taken place in a significant way. There is a
need to develop an appropriate balance between the formal and informal support systems which would guard against over-reliance on
in-home and community-based care, preserve the optimum level of
family support, and prevent exploitation of the family's role by the
formal service system.

4. *What incentives are needed, if any, to preserve and support
family care?*

Since the family is viewed as a key to community maintenance
and cost control, workshop participants generally agreed that the
following incentives are required to bolster the family's natural
caregiving role.

   a. Availability of a comprehensive assessment.
   b. Availability of case management and family counseling ser-
      vices.

c. Availability of a comprehensive range of community, in-home, and institutional long-term care services.
d. Tax credits.

5. *Would expanded coverage of in-home and community-based, long-term care go to a new population rather than substitute for more expensive nursing home care?*

The consensus of the workshop participants was that there is greater need for long-term care services than current and future long-term care systems can bear. Because of the present climate of fiscal stringency, however, it was felt that the system could be structured to emphasize community and in-home care for the narrowly defined population at-risk for nursing home care. This would, in effect, prevent these expanded services from going to a new population.

6. *Is case management an effective approach to controlling the costs of long-term care? What elements of case management are necessary to control costs in service delivery?*

Workshop members felt that case management was an effective mechanism to control long-term care costs by preventing inappropriate service utilization. While the impact and costs of case management services have not been systematically evaluated as part of most ongoing research and demonstration programs, the feeling was that the impact of case management on utilization and client outcomes is more a reflection of the case management process than the additional services provided, or the experimental effect.

The group felt that an effective case management program should include the following elements:

a. gatekeeping (with pre-admission screening and eligibility placement authority),
b. comprehensive assessment,
c. care planning, service arrangement, service coordination, and service monitoring,
d. fiscal control (through budget caps and/or cost-sharing),
e. quality assurance, and
f. advocacy and client/family counseling.

The gatekeeping and financial control elements were viewed by the workshop as most critical to targeting services to the narrow population-at-risk and, at the same time, to holding long-term care costs down.

7. *What should the future long-term care system look like in terms of eligibility, program benefits, covered services, cost sharing, reimbursement, and overall financing methods?*

The group felt that access to the future long-term care system should be based not only on functional disability but also on criteria such as the availability of informal support. Rather than a grant program, it should be an entitlement. Benefits would be provided on an in-kind basis, but experimentation with vouchers and tax credits should not be ruled out. (The potential for abuse was frequently expressed with regard to these two approaches.) Because of the wide variability of need among the impaired elderly population and the potential of downward service substitution, there should be a comprehensive range of community, in-home, and institutional services with a dollar benefit ceiling. When possible, client/family cost-sharing and negotiated flat rates with providers should be used. Overall, the workshop felt that the long-term care component of the Medicare, Medicaid, and Title XX programs should be combined with pooled funding passing through the states to local case management agencies which would perform assessment and arrange for and/or directly deliver some or all needed services.

Summary

In summary, costs are definitely an important consideration in the provision of coordinated community-based services. A good case manager may also have to be a good fiscal manager. Freestanding case management systems such as Triage or ACCESS may provide a fiscally responsible method for organizing case-managed, long-term care systems, since they do not provide services themselves, and thus are not biased towards recommending their own services. They can shop around for the highest quality services provided at the lowest cost assuming more than one agency is available to provide such services. On the other hand, existing providers can play a major role in coordinating and delivering comprehensive long-term care services.

It was felt that a major concern is terminology. When one discusses a dichotomy between informal and formal support, there seems very little disagreement. But the same does not hold true for the supposed dichotomy between institutional services and community-based services. None of us would want to be part of perpetuating stereotypical terminology. For example, in Part II of this volume the outreach programs at the Metropolitan Jewish Geriatric Center in Brooklyn were described. Similar programs are found at the Jewish Home and Hospital for the Aged in Manhattan and also in other long-term care institutions in the city and around the country. These agencies are providing services that, on the one hand, could be called community-based and on the other are delivered from an institutional base. These agencies are composed of a skilled-nursing facility, health-related facility, a certified day care program, and a long-term home health care program, which are certified Medicaid reimbursement programs. Are these services community-based or are they institution-based?

One of the best sites for locating a future coordinated services system for the community may well be the multi-level health care facilities which have already coordinated institutional services. Certainly institutions can act in a fiscally responsible manner. It should be stressed that it is important to distinguish between who should provide the service and who should make decisions about which services are needed. If providers make these care decisions, choices may well be made on the basis of those services that they provide and not strictly on the basis of client need. Thus, an independent agency might be viewed as the most appropriate locus for the assessors and case managers who will have some authority over the providers. If there is fiscal responsibility and it rests with the provider, then there will have to be some means to have them choose the most cost-effective services. Fixed budgets and capitation are examples of such controls. If providers are going to be financially at-risk for choosing a particular service, they will choose a less costly one. In other words, if a provider, nearing bankruptcy, does not already use the most effective method, he would soon learn to use it.

It would seem that the research conducted to date does not offer too many insights into the actual cost and benefit aspect of coordinated services delivery. The "gut" feeling is that these types of programs are beneficial especially as indicated by the Triage program in Connecticut. Further comments about evaluation research appear in the next article.

Reevaluating the Place of Evaluation in Planning for Alternatives to Institutional Care for the Elderly

Barry Gurland
Ruth Bennett
David Wilder

This paper reviews an array of studies evaluating alternative settings and programs for long term care of the elderly. Some major methodological weaknesses of those evaluation studies are reviewed. Substantial ambiguities in the results of those studies are also examined. For both of these reasons, and others, research results have had little impact on policy for long term care of the elderly. The paper argues for an emphasis, in the future, on research that will help provide better information to clients, families, and service providers, rather than on studies aimed at finding which site or model is best for long term care.

Industrial nations have witnessed, in this century, an unprecedented growth in the proportion of elderly in their populations; and the nonindustrial nations can anticipate a similar development in the future (UN General Assembly, Note 1). At the beginning of this century less than 5% of the population of the United States were elderly (65 years of age or older) but this proportion has more than doubled since then and is projected to rise to as much as 14.6% by the year 2020 (National Council on the Aging, 1978). The major factors contributing to this changing demography are increased life expectancy due to control of neonatal and post-partum death rates, and a reduction in the birth rate. In some regions of this country,

Barry Gurland, Ruth Bennett, and David Wilder are affiliated with the Center for Geriatrics and Gerontology, Columbia University, Faculty of Medicine, and New York State Office of Mental Health.

This paper was published in the *Journal of Social Issues,* Volume 37, No. 3, 1981. Reprinted with the permission of the publishers.

such as Florida, migration patterns have already swelled the proportion of elderly to over 16% (N.C.O.A., 1978).

The elderly constitute the large majority (over 92%) of individuals in long term care facilities (LTCF's). The average age of residents in nursing homes in New York State is about 81 years (United States Department of Health, Education and Welfare, 1979). The chance of an elderly person being admitted to a LTCF is over 50 times greater than for a younger person. This heightened risk of institutional admission for the elderly is partly a function of the disability, dependence and other effects of 'age related' chronic disorders, and partly a function of the weak family and community supports that reflect mobility of the family, ageism and the strains of caring for dependent elderly.

There is also some evidence that the elderly with chronic disorders are living longer after the onset of their disability than they did before the introduction of modern methods of management of acute medical crises (Gruenberg, 1978). Increased duration of chronic disorders leads to more of them and to a greater demand for supportive care.

Those individuals who require special care for their chronic health conditions, or who lose their capacity for independent living or acceptable social behavior, and who cannot obtain needed additional health care services, personal assistance or special tolerance in the community, are likely to be admitted to an institution. The rate of institutional admission is highest among the group over 75 years of age. This group is increasing, in absolute size and as a proportion of the general population, faster than even the remainder of the elderly. Furthermore, if current life style patterns continue there is likely to be, in the future, a large increase of single elderly females, especially those who have never married and who may be particularly vulnerable to institutional admission when they become dependent. The never-married are overrepresented about fourfold in nursing homes (U.S.D.H.E.W., 1979).

Thus there are an increasing number of frail and dependent elderly who require long term care from formal and informal support systems. Brady and Masciocchi (1980) see the goal of the long term care system as being "to improve, modify and maintain the optimum level of functions of a disabled target population." Part of the societal response, at least in the USA, has been a proliferation of long term care facilities to provide care and shelter to those elderly who are unable to obtain such services elsewhere. There are over 1

million beds in long term care facilities in the USA, distributed
among some 20,000 institutions, most of which have been established in the past two decades (Butler, 1975). "Homes for the aged
under church auspices had existed for centuries but with the advent
of the Social Security Act [in 1935], a new method of caring for the
elderly . . . other than in county homes . . . evolved. Older people
could suddenly pay for their care in private homes. [However], . . .
the real boom in nursing home care began with Medicare and
Medicaid in 1965" (Linn & Linn, 1980). The growth of this institutional industry has been facilitated, if not actually encouraged, by a
pattern of legislated federal and state funding programs. These programs were, at least initially, responsive to the plight of the frail
elderly person. But they have led to a rising concern about the esca-
lating costs of institutional care, most of which is borne by the
public sector, and about the policy of directing most public funds for
long term care toward institutional rather than non-institutional delivery of care. The public cost of nursing home care has risen faster
than other components of the health care industry. The great majority are operated for profit, in contrast to hospitals of which the great
majority are not-for-profit. Nursing home bed capacity now exceeds
that of hospitals (Linn & Linn, 1980).

The growth of institutions has also led to concerns about the de-
personalization and demoralization of their residents, about the
physical and other abuses to which they may be exposed, and about
relocation stress or transfer trauma (Kasl, 1972). The concerns
about cost and personal well being have turned out to be mutually
reinforcing.

Much effort has gone into attempts to regulate and control the
quality and cost of care given in institutional settings. A thicket of
regulations has sprung up governing rates of reimbursement, standards for structure, organization and staffing, and the types and
degree of disabling conditions which allow admission to institutions.
Monitoring and enforcement procedures operate through a variety
of government bodies at federal and state level as well as through
peer review systems. Yet, the costs of institutional care remain
high, its quality is uncertain and regulatory activities themselves
promote a good deal of dissatisfaction among critics of the institutional system. At its worst, the regulatory system has been blamed
for unjustifiable refusal or relocation of institutional clients, for
wholesale shuffling of residents from mental health institutions to
nursing homes (U.S. Bureau of Census, 1973), for requiring un-

necessary hospitalization of applicants for institutional admission, for overemphasis on the structural characteristics of institutions, paper compliance, process rather than outcome measures of care, and for a general bias towards institutional and medical care rather than other equally important aspects of the spectrum of care.

Non-institutional modes of care for the chronically disabled and frail elderly have always predominated. Even at the apogee of institutional care, far greater numbers of dependent elderly have been supported outside rather than inside of institutions. For every seriously disabled elderly person in a long term care facility in New York City, where institutional beds are relatively numerous, there probably are three equally disabled elderly living at home in the community (Brady, Poulshock, & Masciocchi, 1978; Gurland, Dean, Gurland, & Cook, 1978). The dependent elderly living in the community draw primarily upon the personal assistance of family members, usually a spouse or daughter (Gurland, Copeland, Kuriansky, Kelleher, Sharpe, & Dean, 1981), but may also have access to one or another of a wide variety of formal services provided by public or proprietary agencies. Such services may be provided singly or in aggregates and packages, in the home or in central sites. The various combinations and permutations of services and their delivery sites for the dependent elderly living at home constitute the alternatives to institutional care.

The growth of the nursing home industry has slowed and possibly reversed itself. More and more, the alternatives to institutional care have been seen by planners as reactive to the cost and care problems associated with institutions. Until recently, there was a prevalent and confident expectation that if there were sufficient and adequate alternatives to institutional care, then potential candidates for institutional admission would be diverted to community care programs where they would be less expensively managed, less demoralized, less disengaged and isolated, less depersonalized and less abused than in institutions, and would, in addition, fare better in the course of their physical and mental disorders. In short, it was assumed that alternatives to institutional care would turn out to be cost-effective and also desirable from both humane and public health viewpoints. From this vantage point it was reasonable to assume that many residents of nursing homes could be discharged to less intensive levels of care in the community and new admissions could be reduced as well. Several studies documented the number of elderly who seemed to be misplaced in institutions. The chances of placement in an institution for a given level of disability, may be quite dependent on the state of residence, even where systematic assessment of need for placement is enforced (Foley & Schweider, 1980).

As attention has turned to the alternatives to institutional care, the shortcomings of the alternatives which presently exist have become more evident (Doherty, Segal, & Hicks, 1978). These include: (1) a potentially high demand for these services, from elderly who are not yet and might never be in institutions, that might swamp the existing and planned services without much impact on the number in an institution; (2) difficulty of gaining entry to alternatives of care, given their patchy and often evanescent geographic representation, the maze of rules of eligibility and the inadequacy of information and referral pathways; (3) a lack of well trained staff, hence problems of supervising, monitoring, and regulating against the possibility of fraud, abuse and poor quality care, especially when care is given in such a wide range of sites; (4) high costs of transport for clients to central sites; and high travel time for service providers to peripheral sites; and (5) inefficiencies that are inherent in a system in which clients with multiple problems use multiple services that cut across traditional disciplinary boundaries, where the services are neither coordinated nor integrated. Furthermore, even when the alternative care system is functioning smoothly and efficiently, it may sometimes have the paradoxical effect of hastening rather than delaying a client's admission to an institution (Blenkner, 1967).

It might appear now that the stage has been set for a series of evaluation studies comparing various alternatives of long term care in terms of their benefits and cost-effectiveness and for applying the results of such studies to policy and planning for long term care. In this scenario, the results of the evaluation research would help to determine whether institutional or non-institutional modes of care should be endorsed, and which sectors of these two broad arenas should be encouraged. At a further level of refinement, decisions on the development of services would be based on empirical knowledge about which clients can best be managed in which settings or service programs. However, this paper will seriously question whether policy decisions about alternatives to institutional care can or will be based on results of evaluative studies within the near future.

In presenting a perspective on the role of evaluation research in determining policy on the development of alternatives to institutional care for the elderly we will first describe the current range of alternatives in long term care for the elderly, and the fiscal programs that in large part determine which alternatives remain viable. Then we will consider the methods of evaluation research used in studies of long term care, ambiguities in results of completed studies and the irrelevance of many studies to the process of formulating policy.

CURRENT ALTERNATIVES AND THEIR FISCAL CONTROLS

Range of Alternatives in Long Term Care of the Elderly

There is no useful or clear cut boundary between institutional and non-institutional service models. At the "institutional" end of a spectrum of services lie those that are so organized that almost all aspects of the clients' lives are adjusted to be consistent with the goals of the service organization. These goals in many instances may be unrelated to the best interests of an individual client. At the other end of the spectrum are those services so arranged as to be minimally intrusive and disruptive to the clients' customary mode of existence. There has been a tendency to describe this spectrum as extending along a dimension of restrictiveness: the corresponding policy thrust has been to aim at placing the client in the least restrictive setting compatible with adequate care. However, whereas the concept of institutionality correctly refers to the behavior of the institution, the concept of restrictiveness refers to a variable interaction between the characteristics of the client and those of the institution such that some clients who require a great deal of personal assistance and immediate access to social activities are less restricted in an institution than at home.

Nonetheless, for the purpose of description we can list on the institutional end of the spectrum the geriatric hospital and chronic disease hospital; the extended care, convalescent, and rehabilitation facility; the skilled nursing facility or nursing home, and home for the confused; the long-stay mental hospital and intermediate care or health related facility with or without special mental classification; and hospice. All these facilities provide for patients with severe disorders and disabilities, and, to a greater or lesser extent, emphasize the medical or nursing aspects of care.

Somewhere in the middle of the long term care spectrum are settings that tend to be better related than the facilities described above to the resources and activities of the surrounding community, to have a client population who may or may not be frail but who generally are not severely disabled nor requiring much medical or nursing service, and to be able to provide for the personal and social assistance that many of their clients need. These settings are either alternatives to institutional care, or, if they are regarded as institutions, are considered alternatives to the more intensive levels of care. They include the domiciliary care facility, adult home and proprietary home for adults, the personal care home, the group home, and the congregate care home, enriched housing and the foster home. Further toward the non-institutional end of the spectrum are boarding homes, single room occupancy residential hotels and retirement villages, though some of these settings may have a more disabled client population and acquire some organized health and social services that shift back toward the institutional end of the spectrum.

Definitely on the non-institutional end of the long term care spectrum are services that support the frail elderly person living at home, or with family or friends. Some of these services still have some institutional flavor, in that they are organized in central sites primarily for the sake of efficiency and economy, though the social interaction between attending clients may be an important benefit for them. The central sites include medical clinics, day hospitals and community mental health centers, often with a strong medical orientation; and day care centers, sheltered workshops, luncheon clubs and senior citizen centers, usually with a mainly social orientation. Finally, at the extreme non-institutional end of the spectrum are an array of services that can be delivered into the home. These include: medical house-calls and visiting nurse services; home delivered therapies, such as occupational, speech and physiotherapy; home health aides and health education; housekeeper, home maintenance and laundry services; meals-on-wheels; friendly visiting; regular checking by agencies or mailmen for emergency needs; escort, transport and shopping help; household restructuring; and social services, legal counselling and protective services.

In accordance with convention and legislative custom the alternatives for long term care have been described as a set of categories lying along a care continuum. However, they might better be described as a series of service and care packages varying on multiple dimensions. Thus skilled nursing facilities on the institutional end of the spectrum may provide respite services as part of a home-care program. Conversely, day hospitals serving the community based elderly may share facilities and staff with a skilled nursing facility. Not only do these single components of the long term care system provide an extended range of services spread along the institutional and non-institutional dimension; sets of these components also may be linked into a care complex or system. Such coordinated systems may gain efficiency in various ways. (1) They may offer economies of scale, and economies through sharing of resources, such as when a skilled nursing facility acts also as a health related facility or day hospital. (2) They may offer reductions of unnecessary use of expensive facilities by easing transfer of patients from one to another site for care, as when a geriatric hospital includes an extended care ward or when an intermediate care facility is linked to a home care program. (3) They may provide comprehensive treatment packages that could not be mustered by any one long term care component acting separately. (4) They may offer, through centralization economies of quality and cost control and resource allocations. (5) They may provide advantages, especially preventing excess disability, morbidity and mortality, by tailoring level and type of care to the patients needs rather than letting it be determined by extraneous factors. Long term care must be designed for patients who have multiple problems that extend through and change over time.

Fiscal Programs Directed at Long Term Care of the Elderly

There is a well established body of criticism of the fiscal restraints on the rational development of alternatives to institutional care. A substantial review which is reflected in much of this section is provided by Greenberg and Doth (1980). The most salient attack is on the neglect of potential non-institutional long term care resources by federal funding sources. Federal expenditures for benefits to the elderly exceeded 130 billion dollars in 1980, of which about 33 billion went to Medicare/Medicaid. Of this large category of health care expenditures, only a tiny proportion went to non-institutional long term care (less than 3% of Medicare and about 1% of Medicaid). Even when supplemented by Title XX (Social Security Act) and Title III (Older Americans Act), less than 10% of federal expenditures relevant to long term care are directed at non-institutional services. Moreover, long term care services supported by federal funds are not only primarily institutional but also medical in orientation. This situation, if allowed to continue, could only get worse.

Titles XX and III programs, that promote non-institutional social services, are closed ended.

The provision of an integrated set of community based alternatives to institutional long term care is impeded not only because of limitations on how the federal funds can be used, but also because a number of federal and local funding sources would have to be coordinated in order to muster an array of services that would constitute a core system, or alternative, to institutional care.

The ideology and mechanisms that favor institutional rather than community based alternatives for long term care are widely recognized. *Medicare* has developed as an acute care program. Both its skilled nursing care and its home health care are limited to coverage for 100 days in each benefit period, and a stay in an acute care hospital is a prerequisite. Furthermore, such home care services as are covered under Medicare are targeted at intermittent skilled nursing for medical problems while crucial non-medical services for functionally disabled persons remain uncovered, (e.g., medication, podiatry, perceptual aids and homemaking.) *Medicaid*, based on a means test, covers a wider range of services of value to the elderly with chronic disorders and disability. But the services available, and the income and medical criteria for eligibility, vary widely by state and locality. Although Medicaid home-care benefits do not exclude, as does Medicare, those who have not been in hospital, those who are medically stable, and those who are not housebound, other restrictions and actual practice leaves the program with a heavy institutional bias.

The *Title XX* program has, as one of its major goals, the funding of community based services that prevent inappropriate admission to an institution, (e.g., home makers, congregate meals, transportation, legal services and respite care.) Such services are restricted, on the whole, to those persons earning no more than 115% of the state's median income. *Title III* funds are intended to provide supportive services for those elderly who can thus achieve self-care at home. The services emphasized are home makers, home health aides, home delivered meals, transportation, information and senior citizen centers. The Department of Housing and Urban Development, (*HUD*), provides mortgages, loans and rent subsidies to promote appropriate housing for the elderly and handicapped, including congregate housing. About half of the costs of long term care services for persons outside institutions are borne by patients and families, while public funds support almost all costs of institutional care.

Innovative plans for financing long term care for the elderly include: (1) Proposals to relieve restrictions on the application of existing programs such as Medicare to home care services, especially removal of requirements for prior hospitalization, for having plans endorsed by a physician, and for restricting the range of services, agencies and conditions involved. (2) Proposals for public insurance approaches to long term care, and national health insurance plans, most of which are merely improvements on current programs. (3) Proposals to establish single entry community based care centers that coordinate the delivery of long term care by channelling funds, and assessing, referring and monitoring clients. (4) Proposals to expand the concept of Health Maintenance Organizations to include long term health and social services. Efforts to implement these proposals are being funded, currently, in a makeshift manner by means of demonstration grants. At present, few have been given a secure future. Ostensibly the results of the evaluation of these demonstration projects will determine their continued support.

METHODOLOGICAL PROBLEMS
IN EVALUATING ALTERNATIVES

Identifying the Alternative Modes of Care

Comparison of the functioning of alternatives requires that the essential characteristics of each alternative be explicit so that the differences between the alternatives are clear and differences in the results can be related to them. But conventional categories of services and sites are heterogeneous. Alternatives that are placed by conventional labels into the same category (e.g., skilled nursing facility) might in fact provide quite dissimilar arrays of services. Conversely, apparently different labels may nevertheless refer to similar types of services (e.g., a skilled nursing facility in the United States and a geriatric hospital in England).

A multidimensional approach to the description of alternatives in long term care can be more precise than a categorical description. Each service unit can be described in terms of its physical structure and technology, neighborhood setting, administration, number of personnel, and their training type and mix of client problems, availability of personal, medical and social services, costs and mode of reimbursement, and the like. However, these more or less structural properties say less than do the dynamic aspects of a service about the quality of care received by clients in a given setting, or about how a system of care operates. Among the important dynamic aspects of a care setting are its manner of: selecting clients; effecting their transitions into the system and between its components; conducting interactions between staff and patients; of relating to the surrounding community; and deferring to the preferences of the clients. Other, sometimes elusive, dynamic aspects are: the explicit and covert goals of the administrators of the service unit; the efforts expended in securing the future of the service; and, abuses that occur within the system. Unfortunately, the structural features of modes of care are more frequently documented than are the dynamic aspects which may require subtle and laborious assessment procedures.

Matching Patients Across Institutions and Their Alternatives

When patients are randomly assigned to treatment settings it is often assumed that the patient groups are comparable between settings with respect to characteristics that may affect outcomes. Post hoc analyses are needed to assess the degree to which observed characteristics of the patient groups justify that assumption of comparability. Comparisons between alternatives within a single system of care, or within a limited geographic region, can sometimes be based on a design for random assignment of patients, though they often are not so designed.

In comparisons of systems of care in widely separated geographic regions, random assignment of patients is usually out of the question. Investigators must rely on quasi-experimental designs, involving matching patients between treatment settings, and must be aware of their limitations (Cook & Campbell, 1979). Two classes of characteristics are especially germane: (1) baseline measures of initial severity of health or social problems; and (2) prognostic features that affect rates of decline or recovery irrespective of initial severity (e.g., type of problem; premorbid level of function). There are a variety of assessment procedures that can serve these ends, including measures of basic and instrumental activities of living, morale and affective state, cognitive function, social activities and contacts, objective and subjective health, and operationally defined diagnoses. Unfortunately, even these relatively straightforward procedures may vary, unexpectedly, between treatment settings. Similar patients may not obtain similar scores when placed in different settings in which different other variables are operating.

Recording Extraneous Events Affecting Outcome

Clients of a long term care service do not exist only within that service; they are exposed to environmental influences that extend far beyond. For that matter, the service itself exists within a larger political and societal context and has a history of its own. Events and situations extraneous to the patients' condition and the treatment service may alter the outcome of treatment. The most important extraneous influences to consider would include: stressful life events such as bereavements; acts such as encouragement and advice by members of the patients' social networks; receipt of treatment from additional sources; changes in national or local policy; turnover of staff; the stage of development of the treatment setting (e.g., whether the program is new, seasoned or winding down); and the expectations of the evaluation team if they are not blind to the nature of the evaluation and treatment received by the participating parties. There is little possibility of avoiding or keeping constant all events or situations, nor are such events often recorded and considered in evaluation studies.

Determining the Appropriate Goals of Long Term Care

The most pertinent criterion for evaluating alternatives in long term care is the effectiveness of these alternatives in achieving certain outcome goals, including: securing, for the functionally impaired elderly person, whatever personal assistance, basic care and shelter is required and is not available from informal or other formal sources; enhancement of survival, functioning and social engagement levels as much as possible for that person (Bloom, 1975); and doing so while preserving as far as possible the continuity of the person's life style and a high state of morale.

While all of these are generally acknowledged to be important, there may be considerable variation in the emphasis placed on these various outcome goals by various components of long term care systems. Those components at the institutional end of the spectrum, or those espousing a medical and nursing model of treatment, may stress the preservation or improvement of functioning; while components at the other end of the spectrum may focus on the quality of life of their clients.

Cost containment goals are also regarded as crucial goals for long term care alternatives in the current politico-economic view of a society with limited resources. Fullerton (Note 2) probably reflects the majority opinion of planners when he states that a ceiling for long term care expenditures is not only likely but necessary in order to control costs. This view has, perhaps more than any other, motivated contemporary evaluation studies of long term care. Kalish (1980) remarks that "only very recently has the cost-effectiveness literature [on long term care] of the elderly begun to deal with the value of life satisfaction, pleasure, and enjoyment. It is difficult to integrate these factors into the cost-effective equation in a quantitative fashion but it makes a travesty of the concept of effectiveness if they are omitted."

So far we have restricted the selection of goals to those that emerge from the 'raison d'être' of the care system. However, quite different goals may be equally important in shaping the nature and utilization of the long term care system: the desire of a service to perpetuate itself; the striving for identity and purposefulness on the part of the administrators and staff; the perceptions and preferences about fulfillment of needs held by the clients, their families, or their neighbors; the competing interests of other services or other clients; and the conservation of personal as opposed to public resources. Obvious difficulties can arise in an evaluation study in documenting and reconciling these various perspectives with their differing and sometimes conflicting goals.

USE OF EVALUATION STUDY RESULTS IN POLICY ON LONG TERM CARE

The many methodological problems of studies evaluating alternatives in long term care of the elderly would lead one to expect that the results of such studies would be inconsistent and ambiguous, and thus they would not produce results that would be sufficiently definitive enough to override other considerations in deciding policy. Review of some demonstration projects and comparative studies in this arena confirms that expectation.

An evaluation of the Wisconsin Community Care Organization (Applebaum, Seidl, & Austin, 1980) was inconclusive, despite ran-

dom assignment of applicants to experimental and other services only after they had met a criterion (on the GFRS scale) of need for
institutional care. Biases were found in the way in which the GFRS
was administered; differences were found between experimental
subjects and those referred before and after the experimental period;
and CCO services were not even delivered to a large number of the
designated experimental group members. Analysis of the Monroe
County Long Term Care Program, ACCESS, after the initial 24
months of activity (Eggert, Bowlyow, & Nichols, 1980) depended
on a comparison of that program to results in six other counties in
New York, on variables such as: number of patients in acute care
hospitals awaiting admission to nursing homes; relative changes in
beneficiaries; costs per beneficiary; and other costs. All of these
comparisons may be misleading for a variety of reasons. The
evaluators cautioned that comparison groups cannot be confidently
constructed on the assessment of need for institutional care because
of contextual biases in the assessments. The evaluators of the community based single entry system in Connecticut, TRIAGE, that
used Medicare waivers, (Hicks, Quinn, Segal, & Raisz, 1980) reported a statistically significant difference between the deceased
group and the total population on six of seven key variables and between the withdrawn/terminated group and the total population in
their program on two of seven variables. In addition, a non-equiva-
lent comparison group was studied using a quasi-experimental
design and seven different modes of statistical analysis, but un-
anticipated differences were found between these samples as well,
and basic questions about study results remained unanswered
despite sophisticated statistical analysis. Weissert, Wan, Livieratos,
and Katz (1980) reported a comparison of clients randomly assigned
to adult *day care centers* with strong health care components, and a
control group using Medicaid waivers, in four cities. Twenty-five
percent of the experimental group did not use the day services that
were provided, only small proportions of the experimental and control groups entered nursing homes during the follow-up year, and
costs for the day care group were considerably higher than for the
controls. After conducting sophisticated statistical tests the authors
concluded that day care had few beneficial effects. Hammill and
Oliver (1975) carried out an evaluation of a day hospital at Burke
Rehabilitation Center, randomly assigning patients with chronic ill-
nesses and physical disabilities to the day hospital or back to the
community. They had a nine month followup. Results were incon-

sistent across different outcome measures, and staff ratings were not blind to the study design and subject disposition.

The results of these evaluation studies do not show dramatic differences between the outcomes of the alternatives in long term care. The Congressional Budget Office's report (U.S. Congress, 1977) on one large scale demonstration project (albeit premature in the view of Blum & Minkler, 1980) discounted the findings reported at that stage on the grounds that they were either of questionable or limited generalizability and value! Doherty and Hicks (1975) criticize cost-effectiveness comparisons of day care centers because they are marred by lack of standardization of assessment procedures, including those for determining the costs of care. Wolf (1980) believes that ''because concepts are complex and difficult to define and measure, most intervention studies [of alternatives to institutional care for the elderly] have not been conclusive.''

If the question for evaluation is whether one form of care is generally more cost-effective than another, then the answer is decidedly ambiguous. The question might be differently framed: If an alternative in long term care is valued for personal or societal reasons should it be discouraged because it is comparatively too costly and ineffective? None of the alternatives in the spectrum considered here can be absolutely disqualified for all classes of persons or disorders on these grounds.

A movement away from comparison of unrelated sites of care to comparisons of systems of care recognizes that all components of a care continuum have a useful function. Above all a variety of components provides *options* for the client, for the family, and for health care professionals. Providing options is a rational response to uncertainty about the therapeutic, moral and financial strengths and weaknesses of the various alternatives. This is even more the case because such uncertainties are compounded by the need for a fit between particular subgroups of clients and the long term care system.

It is unreasonable to expect that any alternative now established in the long term care system will disappear in the foreseeable future. Further evaluative research is not likely to have much impact on the viability or growth of any now established alternative. Rossman and Burnside (1975) conclude that ''home care services have been honored more in the breech than the observance despite excellent demonstrations of their usefulness.'' There is no parallel here with drug research in which exacting controls over selection of patients and administration of a drug can provide broadly generalized information on the relative benefits and side-effects of alternative drugs. Even under these circumstances, only the most dramatic results can compete with other factors determining use of drugs.

It must also be noted that some studies are restricted to comparisons of treated and untreated groups, rather than groups treated in various treatment modalities. This approach to evaluation is intended to be analagous to the design of a drug-placebo study, but the analogy may be spurious. The difference between active and placebo ingredients in drugs is a great deal clearer than it is in long term care; and the progression of specification of the mechanism of a drug's effect is quite different from the evolution of a long term care service. A more appropriate analogy would be to studies designed to distinguish the specific and non-specific effects of psychotherapy. These do not necessarily involve comparisons between treated and untreated groups.

The factors likely to shape the future system of alternatives in long term care will be the relative power of provider and consumer constituencies and the total resources available for health care. These factors will determine arrangements by reinforcing or suppressing supportive attitudes toward the aged person, frailty and dependence, individual and family rights, medical and social or personal care models, technological or moral solutions, and institutional or non-institutional settings.

Maddox (1980) points to several factors influencing policy on alternatives to institutional care that go beyond, or perhaps not as far as, information on the comparative costs and effectiveness of these alternatives: non-institutional care shifts much of the burden of costs from the public to the private sector; removing patients from institutional settings reduces the risk of high cost interventions involving intensive technology; the need for the freedom of choosing between alternatives; a cultural preference for asserting familial responsibility for older persons; and a positive image associated with the 'curative' short-stay hospital in contrast to a negative attitude toward long term institutions. However, the overriding appeal to the public of high technology medicine gives Maddox serious pause: ". . . , it is not at all clear that either (health care providers or consumers) would respond affirmatively to more non-institutional care if this meant fewer hospital beds, rationed access to hospitals and physicians, or reduction in the specialized test and therapeutic procedures that are in the heart of contemporary diagnosis.''

It may be that demand for some options will exceed supply even when the main determinant of demand is the client's and family's informed choice. It is tempting to resolve the allocation of scarce resources, primarily by choosing the most cost-effective fit between the potential clients and alternative care options (Dovenmuhle, 1971; Kahana, 1973; Lawton, 1970; Sherwood, Morris, & Barnhart, 1975; Tobin, Hammerman, & Rector, 1972). However, this approach may turn into a game of musical chairs in which some clients get no options or resources at all; for example, programs that require clients to meet a criterion for the risk of being institutionalized. Furthermore, approaches of this nature, given the ambiguity of research results, may turn out to be evanescent: it is a contemporary but not necessarily enduring article of faith that keeping people out of institutions is a rationale for a continuum of care.

It is hardly likely that more refined instruments or more ingenious research designs will produce the dramatic contrasts we do not now have between alternative sites and models for long term care.

The future role of evaluation research should be to improve the information available to consumers on what they can personally expect from specific alternatives, to providers on what they can do better for specific clients, and to policy makers on ways and costs of improving the system. Wolf (1980) states that "appropriate placement has become a central theme in long term care. The underlying assumption is that the better the fit between the individual and the level of service received, the more likely that the desired outcomes will be achieved." He calls for better specification of the environmental and service arrangements that promote optimal functioning of clients. The pathway to these ends is through a focus on the fit between the individual and the continuum of long term care.

There have been historical cycles of bias in favor of or against institutional care. We are just now emerging from the latter phase in which it was taken for granted that keeping the elderly out of institutions was a desirable goal subsuming a larger set of secondary goals for the optimization of the quality of life and functioning of the elderly person. Stereotypes, societal values and politico-economic motives probably have had more to do with producing an anti-institutional bias than has empirical evidence regarding the secondary goals mentioned above. We are left with some evaluation studies in which the criterion of a successful outcome for an alternative in long term care is mainly the avoidance of admission to an institution of an elderly person who is presumed to be at risk for such admission.

The most challenging research issue is *not* whether non-institutional alternatives are as effective as institutional care, but rather whether it is feasible, within the resources available, to provide every client with a full range of options for care together with good advice as to what the various options can offer to client and family (e.g., in terms of services, quality of life and outcomes). Several of the studies reported speak to this question. Increasing the options for care through removal of reimbursement restrictions does not necessarily lead to spiralling costs. The coordination of multiple services, diverse agents, and alternative sites can be achieved through policy organization, and consolidation of authority over finances and monitoring care.

One possible reason that evaluation studies of alternatives in long term care give ambiguous results is their focus on heterogeneous groups of clients and treatments within programs. If good advice is to be offered to clients and families reviewing the options for care then much more precision about client type, treatment and outcomes is required in identifying which clients will do best in which programs. Perhaps, out of such precision, could come more striking contrasts in cost-effectiveness between alternatives than now exist.

REFERENCE NOTES

1. U.N. General Assembly. *The question of aging and the aged.* Unpublished report presented by the Secretary General. United Nations, 1971.
2. Fullerton, W. D. *Finding the money and paying for long term care services—the devil's briarpatch.* Paper prepared for symposium on long term care policy options. Williamsburg, Virginia, July 11-13, 1980.

REFERENCES

Applebaum, R., Seidl, F. W., & Austin, C. D. The Wisconsin community care organization: Preliminary findings from the Milwaukee experiment. *The Gerontologist,* 1980, *20*(3), 350-355.

Blenkner, M. Environment change and the aging individual. *The Gerontologist,* 1967, 101-105.

Bloom, M. Evaluation instruments: Tests and measurements in long term care. In S. Sherwood (Ed.) *Long term care: A handbook for researchers, planners and practitioners.* New York: Spectrum, 1975, 573-627.

Blum, S. R., & Minkler, M. Toward a continuum of caring alternatives: Community based care for the elderly. *Journal of Social Issues,* 1980, *36*(2), 133-152.

Brady, S. J., & Masciocchi, C. Data for long-term care planning by health systems agencies. *American Journal of Public Health,* 1980, *70*(11), 1194-1198.

Brady, S. J., Poulshock, S. W., & Masciocchi, C. The family caring unit: A major consideration in the long-term support system. *The Gerontologist,* 1978, *18*(6), 556-561.

Butler, R. *Why survive: On growing old in America.* New York: Harper & Row, 1975.

Cook, T. D., & Campbell, D. T. *Quasi-experimentation: Design and analysis issues for field settings.* Chicago, IL: Rand McNally College Publishing Co., 1979.

Doherty, N., & Hicks, B. The use of cost-effectiveness analysis in geriatric day care. *The Gerontologist,* 1975, *15,* 412-417.

Doherty, N., Segal, J., & Hicks, B. Alternatives to institutionalization for the aged: Viability and cost-effectiveness. *Aged Care and Services Review,* 1978, *1*(1).

Dovenmuhle, R. V. Locus of care: Decision making in relation to individual need and available alternatives. In A. G. Feldman (Ed.) *Community mental health and aging.* Los Angeles, CA: USC Gerontology Center, 1971.

Eggert, G. M., Bowlyow, J. E., & Nichols, C. W. Gaining control of the long term care system: First returns from the Access experiment. *The Gerontologist,* 1980, *20*(3), 356-363.

Foley, W. J., & Schweider, D. P. A comparison of the level of care predictions of six long-term care patient assessment systems. *American Journal of Public Health,* 1980, *70,* 1152-1161.

Greenberg, J., & Doth, D. An essay in financing long term care. In *Selected topics in long term care,* AOA Contract No., HEW-105-79-3008. Elm Associates, 1980.

Gruenberg, E. Epidemiology. In R. Katzman, R. D. Terry, & K. L. Bick (Eds.) *Alzheimers disease: Senile dementia and related disorders,* (Aging, vol. 7). New York: Raven Press, 1978, 323-326.

Gurland, B., Copeland, J., Kuriansky, J., Kelleher, M., Sharpe, L., & Dean, L. *The mind and mood of aging.* New York: The Haworth Press, 1981.

Gurland, B., Dean, L., Gurland, R., & Cook, D. Personal time dependency in New York city: Findings from the U.S.—U.K. Cross-national geriatric community study. In *Dependency in the elderly of New York City: Report of a research utilization workshop.* New York: Community Council of Greater New York, 1978.

Hamill, C. M., & Oliver, R. C. *Final report: The day hospital: An alternative to institutionalization.* Administration on Aging. Grant No. 93-P-75203/203, 1975.

Hicks, B. C., Quinn, J., Segal, J., & Raisz, H. (Eds.) *Triage: Coordinated delivery of services to the elderly.* Final report—National center for health services research. Grant No. HSO2563, 1980.

Kahana, E. The human treatment of old people in institutions. *The Gerontologist,* 1973, *13,* 282-290.

Kalish, R. A. *An essay, in adult day care services: An introduction to the literature,* AOA contract No. HEW-105-79-3008, Elm Associates, 1980.

Kasl, S. Physical and mental health effects of involuntary relocation and institutionalization on the elderly—A review. *American Journal of Public Health,* 1972 (62), 377-384.

Lawton, M. P. Assessment, integration and environments for older people. *The Gerontologist,* 1970, *10,* 38-46.

Linn, W., & Linn, B. Qualities of institutional care that affect outcome. *Aged Care and Services Review,* 1980, *2*(3).

Maddox, G. L. The continuum of care: Movement toward the community. In Ewald W. Busse, & Dan G. Blazer (Eds.) *Handbook of geriatric psychiatry.* New York: Reinhold Co., 1980.

National Council on the Aging, Inc. *Fact book on aging: A profile of America's older population,* 1978.

Rossman, I., & Burnside, I. M. The United States of America. In J. C. Brocklehurst (Ed.) *Geriatric care in advanced societies,* (chap. 4). Baltimore, MD: University Park Press, 1975, 85-112.

Sherwood, S., Morris, J. N., & Barnhart, E. Developing a system for assigning individuals into an appropriate residential setting. *Journal of Gerontology,* 1975, *30,* 331-342.

Tobin, S. S., Hammerman, J., & Rector, V. Preferred disposition of institutionalized aged. *The Gerontologist,* 1972.

U.S. Bureau of Census. Census of population: 1970 Subject reports. *Persons in institu-*

tions and other group quarters, final report. PC (2)-4E. Washington D.C.: U.S. General Printing Office, 1973.

U.S. Congress. Congressional budget office. *Long term care for the elderly and disabled.* Budget House paper. Washington, D.C.: U.S. Government Printing Office, August, 1977.

U.S. Department of Health Education and Welfare. *The national nursing home survey: 1977 Summary for the United States,* Publication No. 79-1794, July, 1979.

Weissert, W. G., Wan, T., Livieratos, B., & Katz, S. Effects and costs of day care services for the chronically ill: A randomized experiment. *Medical Care,* 1980, *18*(6), 567-584.

Wolf, R. S. Appropriate placement and long-term care health planning. *American Journal of Public Health,* 1980, *70*(11), 1144-1145.

Part IV
CONCLUSIONS

Concluding Remarks

Ruth Bennett
Susana Frisch
Barry Gurland
David Wilder

In the previous chapters some of the highly complex aspects of the long-term care system have been discussed and different models of service delivery have been described.

New York State is fortunate to have so many demonstrations to inform its ultimate long-term care policy and system. It will be interesting to see what sort of long-term care system evolves in the future. Clearly, the state cannot afford to expand the nursing home sector. On the other hand, nursing homes are involved in the community-based demonstration programs and may have within them the most experienced personnel from a professional and fiscal management point of view.

Presumably the results of all of the demonstrations will be compared and contrasted in order to develop a viable long-term care system in New York State. It is unfortunate that no two demonstrations used the same methods and measures of evaluation. Nonetheless there are not so many diverse measures available and in use so that there will be considerable overlap in the resulting data. Probably New York State will need to retain a variety of community-based models if it is to hold to its policy of allowing localities to determine how they will serve their frail elderly and support informal support systems. It would be regrettable if the successful demonstration programs were not incorporated into an ongoing New York State long-term care system. Certainly the clients served by the demonstrations will need to be absorbed by some sort of permanent long-term care system if they are not to be institutionalized when the demonstrations end, which most are scheduled to do by mid 1983 or in 1984. The CASA program seems also to be developing as a demonstration program. Will it win out in the competition for which model will be promoted as the statewide model? Or will localities be encouraged and supported to develop their own models? Will the CASA program be able to absorb the clients of the other demonstrations which are ending or will the CASA demonstrations also end leaving many unserved clients?

It will be interesting to see what is developed for the near-Medicaid level clients who are too poor to purchase needed services but not poor enough to receive them from Medicaid. Certainly, future long-term care policy should be addressed to them. It is hoped a two class system will not evolve in long-term care in which the rich will be able to purchase nursing home services while the poor will have to use the alternative system. Presumably there will be mechanisms to insure a mix of clients in both systems. As long as the alternative systems are geared chiefly to Medicaid level clients such a mix is not possible. Competition probably should be encouraged to develop the best model or models for particular localities. The role for the state might remain regulatory and supportive. However, it is not yet clear what role New York State will play.

Nonetheless, it should be clear that New York State is grappling with complex long-term care issues which are confronting all of the states in the nation. What sort of policy and system emerges in New York will undoubtedly be of interest to all of the states, many of whom are also experimenting with a variety of long-term care system models. Clearly a statewide policy and system need to be developed very soon because the costs of clients backed up in acute care hospitals cannot be afforded nor is there a likelihood of increasing nursing home beds.

It is hoped that the issues discussed in this volume will contribute to the development of a comprehensive long-term care policy and system in New York State.

Suggested Issues
for Further Discussion

Ruth Bennett
Susana Frisch
Barry Gurland
David Wilder

A number of issues remain which did not receive much attention at this meeting but which, perhaps, can be addressed at subsequent meetings. These issues are as follows:

(1) What can we learn from the traditional home delivered services as compared to the model programs? For example, the Home Attendant Program of New York City is a traditional program which serves about 25,000 people. One of the problems is that attendants receive minimal training. Not much is known about the quality of care delivered, about patients' characteristics, nor about the kind of services delivered. It is a huge program about which very few data exist. It is assumed that many of the patients, at least the ones getting 24-hour care, would have to be institutionalized if the home attendant program were not available. The National Home Care Council has conducted several national surveys on homemaker services. The Department of Labor is predicting a great shortage of workers as the need for home care grows. It becomes more and more difficult to attract good people into this kind of work because of poor pay, lack of a career ladder, and lack of status. There is concern whether there will be enough women (or men) who will want to care either for relatives at home or work at this sort of job in the future. Unless the agencies can find a way to upgrade the work and pay, it is going to become harder to find people who will want to be attendants in either institutional or community-based programs. Currently these workers are mostly women, and many of them in many parts of the country are minority women; thus, issues of sexism and racism are inevitably involved.

In order to evaluate the home care demonstrations it is important to understand which types of patient and which types of services are involved and to differentiate the homemaker program, the traditional homecare program, and the demonstration long-term health care programs. There seems to be a tremendous overlap which will have to be more clearly understood. Assuming uniformity of units of service may be fallacious. One cannot assume that one type of service given to one client by one agency is equivalent to a similar type of service delivered to another client by a different provider.

(2) Another important area requiring further attention is the issue of what kinds of agencies are best suited to provide community-based, long-term care. As was previously mentioned, traditional home attendant and home care programs have been providing this care for years. However, there is concern over whether or not these programs are delivering comparable services. This raises a further question of how one achieves a balance between public and non-public agencies involved in long-term care system reform. This raises a critical issue particularly in view of the fact that many voluntary agencies currently are experiencing severe financial problems and are possibly looking to redefine their mission in the communities they serve. Although these programs have the expertise and resources, whether they are community based or institution based, government has a major role to play in the system reform because it is funding the demonstrations. However the important question of how to achieve a balance should be raised and debated publicly.

(3) The role of gatekeeping is another important issue. A person doing the gatekeeping or the assessment or the referral will be given a budget that he must stay within, and this will be the controlling factor for decision making. Although a number of models for service mix and delivery are available, financial responsibility remains the prime factor, and no model can function without that restraint. Possibly, the public or governmental sector could be involved in setting a minimum set of standards and act in a regulatory capacity, as they have done in the past. Although in one of the models previously described, government agencies were doing the gatekeeping, in most cases government would not be directly involved in the gatekeeping functions. However, it has been suggested that such a system should be public with an advisory board representing all sectors of the service system.

In a draft paper entitled "Long Term Care Policy Options" (March 1981), Donald Schneider makes some observations about what the literature suggests. These observations include statements like "providers cannot coordinate" or "providers cannot be gate-keepers." Schneider mentions a paper written by Callahan in which he argued that a human service agency which is providing services could not coordinate other agencies in the community. However, it should be pointed out that more recently Callahan has become the advocate of the social health maintenance organization which does lodge the gatekeeping function with a provider who also channels services. A second point made in the Schneider paper is that there must be strong public involvement. As mentioned earlier, it would be foolish to suggest that the government abstain from playing a major role when it pays a major part of the bill, but looking at long-term care system development in this country, it is evident that the major innovators and risk takers have been the freestanding voluntary agencies who are service providers. If they were good enough to develop most long-term care experiments in the first place, are they not good enough to continue the system?

(4) The role of the case manager is another issue for consideration. The New York City Human Resources Administration (HRA), based upon a New York State Department of Social Services (DSS) directive, has always maintained that it is acting as the case manager for the long-term home health care program. Several voluntary long-term home health care programs in New York City have challenged that notion. They maintain that the case manager is that individual who conducts the primary part of the assessment and has 24-hour responsibility for the case and for meeting a client's needs. Furthermore, the case manager's agency is at risk of losing its license if it does something wrong and is also at financial risk if it exceeds the negotiated costs for the plan of care. In a sense, the case manager carries the beeper and can be beeped in the middle of the night to take care of a client's problem. While it is currently understood that New York City HRA is the case manager for the home health program, the reality is that they are the gatekeepers, and this is a political issue which has to be addressed. A political analysis of the community-based coordinated service systems might be a valuable contribution to the field.

The papers in Part III describe case management as a complex set of functions and case managers as a certain breed of professionals within the coordinated service delivery system. It is important to view these elements within the context of their usefulness in the overall purpose of improving the quality of care for the elderly. It also seems unfortunate that at this particular point in time too strong an emphasis is put on cost containment as part of case management. Although cost containment is always the constraint within which any innovations and developments occur and has to be contended with as a reality of life, it is certainly not the main reason for the development of what is obviously intended to be an improvement in the nature of services and the way the elderly can relate to their services. If case managers are merely going to be a new kind of bookkeeper, then we may be inviting demoralization of that profession at the outset. Hopefully, what is intended is a new method for delivering long-term care in the community resulting in better utilization of resources and improved care.

A number of other interesting issues ranging from mere descriptions of current procedures to searching questions about underlying processes were raised. Some of the questions seem to require very lengthy answers and further thought, such as: How to serve people who are not immediately at risk for institutionalization? How to identify people who really are at risk for immediate institutional care? How to avoid dependency-fostering in case management? How to deal with the multiplicity of assessment instruments and methods for different purposes? Which clients can be served more efficiently by a cheaper method? How does one avoid erosion of informal supports?

Many fascinating issues remain to be considered. It is not uncommon that a conference such as this one ends with more questions than answers, and participants come away with many unresolved problems to think through. It is hoped that future workshops can be organized by interested professionals who want to continue to deal with these issues and work out solutions to the problems. And perhaps later on another conference could be convened at which time the results and benefits of the workshops could be shared with a wider audience.

APPENDICES

Recommended Readings

ABT Associates Inc. *Methodology for Finding, Classifying and Comparing Costs for Services in Long-Term Care Settings*, Manual and Executive Summary, January 1977.

Beatrice, D. "Case Management: A Policy Option for Long Term Care," in J. J. Callahan, Jr. and S. S. Wallack (eds.), *Reforming the Long Term Care System*. Lexington, Mass.: D. C. Heath and Company, 1981.

Bennett, R. and Wilder, D. "Innovation without Followthrough: A Study of Nursing Home Experiences," in J. E. O'Brien and N. A. Whitelaw (eds.), *Apathy in America: An Assessment of Care for the Neglected Elderly*. New York: Sage Publishing Co., 1980.

Bennett, R., Killeffer, E., and Wilder, D. Executive Summary of Final Report on "Characteristics of Institutions Successful in Promoting Innovative Programs for the Aged" (AoA Grant Number OHD-AoA-90-AR-0005), February 1983 (manuscript).

Branch, L. G., Callahan, J. J. Jr., and Jette, A. "Targeting Home Care Services to Vulnerable Elders: Massachusetts Home Care Corporation." *Home Health Care Services Quarterly*, Summer 1981, 2(2), 41.

Branch, L. G. and Jette, A. M. "Prospective Study of Long-Term Care Institutionalization Among the Aged." *American Journal of Public Health*, 1982, 72, 1373-1379.

Callahan, J. J. Jr. "A Systems Approach to Long Term Care," in J. J. Callahan, Jr. and S. S. Wallack (eds.), *Reforming the Long Term Care System*. Lexington, Mass.: D. C. Heath and Company, 1981.

Department of Health and Human Services. The Federal Council on the Aging. "The Need for Long Term Care: Information and Issues." *A Chartbook of the Federal Council on the Aging*, DHHS Publication No. (OHDS) 81-20704, 1981.

Diamond, L. M. and Berman, D. E. "The Social/Health Maintenance Organization: A Single Entry, Prepaid, Long Term Care Delivery System," in J. J. Callahan, Jr. and S. S. Wallack (eds.), *Reforming the Long Term Care System*. Lexington, Mass.: D. C. Heath and Company, 1981.

Eggert, G. M., Bowlyow, J. E., and Nichols, C. W. "Gaining Control of the Long Term Care System: First Returns from the ACCESS Experiment." *The Gerontologist*, 1980, 20(3), 356-363.

Estes, C. L. "Community Planning for the Elderly: A Study of Goal Displacement." *Journal of Gerontology*, 1974, 29, 684-691.

Estes, C. L. *The Aging Enterprise*. San Francisco: Jossey-Bass, 1979.

Estes, C. L. "Barriers to Effective Community Planning for the Elderly." *The Gerontologist*, 1973, 13, 173-181.

Etzioni, A. *Modern Organizations*. Englewood Cliffs, N.J.: Prentice-Hall, 1964.

"Facing an Aging Society." Seminar presented at the Swedish Consulate (U.S. and Canadian sections), New York City, October 1978.

Gottesman, L. E., Isizaki, B., and MacBride, S. M. "Service Management: Concepts and Models." *The Gerontologist*, August 1979, 19(4), 378.

Gurland, B., Kuriansky, J., Sharpe, L., Simon, R., Stiller, P., and Birkett, P. "The Comprehensive Assessment and Referral Evaluation (CARE)—Rationale development and reliability. Part II, a Factor Analysis." *International Journal of Aging and Human Development*, 1977, 8, 9-42.

Harvard Club of New York. *Long Term Home Health Care in New York State: The Experience of the Lombardi Program to Date*. Report of the Symposium, June 2, 1980.

The Health Care Financing Administration. *Research and Demonstrations in Health Care Financing 1980-81.*

Hedrick, S. C., Katz, S., and Stroud, M. W. III. "Patient Assessment in Long Term Care: Is There a Common Language?" *Aged Care and Services Review,* 1980-81, *2*(4), 1, 3-19.

ICF Incorporated. *Formulation of an Actuarial Cost Model for Federal Long-Term Care Programs,* Final Report and Executive Summary, September 30, 1982.

Jones, E. W. et al. *Patient Classification for Long Term Care: User Manual,* DHEW Publication No. HRA 75-3107, DHEW, Health Resources Administration, Bureau of Health Services Research and Evaluation, 1974.

Kane, R. L. and Kane, R. A. "Alternatives to Institutional Care of the Elderly: Beyond the Dichotomy." *The Gerontologist,* 1980, *20,* 249-259.

Kane, R. L. and Kane, R. A. *Assessing the Elderly: A Practical Guide to Measurement.* Lexington, Mass.: D. C. Heath, 1981.

Kane, R. L., Bell, R., Riegler, S., Wilson, A., and Kane, R. A. "Assessing the Outcomes of Nursing Home Patients." *The Gerontologist,* in press.

Kane, R. L. and Kane, R. A. "Care of the Aged: Old Problems in Need of New Solutions." *Science,* 1978, *200,* 913.

Kane, R. L., Bell, R., Riegler, S., Wilson, A., and Keeler, E. "Predicting the Outcomes of Nursing Home Patients." *The Gerontologist,* in press.

Kane, R. L. and Kane, R. A. (eds.) *Values and Long-Term Care.* Lexington, Mass.: D. C. Heath, 1982.

Katz, S., Ford, A. F., Moskowitz, R. W., Jackson, B. A., and Jaffee, M. W. "Studies of Illness in the Aged. The Index of ADL: A Standardized Measure of Biological and Psychosocial Function." *Journal of the American Medical Association,* 1963, *185,* 94.

Kethley, A. J. and Herriott, M. "Jointly-used elderly client data in mental health and aging programs: Implications for mental health service." Presented at the 33rd Annual Meeting of the Gerontological Society of America, San Diego, California, November 1980.

Kole, D. M. Testimony before the Mental Health Subcommittee of the Senate Committee on Social and Health Services on Geriatric Mental Health Services, Highline-West Seattle Community Mental Health Center, 1979.

Lawton, M. P. and Brody, E. "Assessment of Older People: Self-Maintaining and Instrumental Activities of Daily Living." *The Gerontologist,* 1969, *9,* 179-188.

Lawton, M. P. "Assessing the Competence of Older People," in D. Kent, R. Kastenbaum, and J. Sherwood (eds.), *Research, Planning and Action for the Elderly.* New York: Behavioral Publications, 1972.

Lawton, M. P., Moss, M., Fulcomer, M., and Kleban, M. H. "A Research and Service Oriented Multi-level Assessment Instrument." *Journal of Gerontology.* 9, 1982, *37,* 91-99.

Mathematica Policy Research, Inc. *The National Long Term Care Demonstration Program.* Princeton, N.J., 1981 (an unpublished report).

Meltzer, J., Farrow, F., and Richman, H. *Policy Options in Long-Term Care.* Chicago: University of Chicago Press, 1981.

Mendelsohn, M. A. *Tender Loving Greed.* New York: Alfred A. Knopf, 1974.

Morris, R. "Coordinating Services for the Elderly: The Promise and Limits of Coordinating Health, Mental Health, and Social Services." Prepared for the Regional Meetings on the Coordination of Services for Children and the Elderly, 1980.

Orlans, H. (ed.) *Human Services Coordination,* A panel report and accompanying papers on four regional meetings. Published by The Council of State Governments and the National Academy of Public Administration. Lexington, Kentucky, 1982.

Pfeiffer, E. "Psychopathology and social pathology," in J. Birren and J. W. Schaie, (eds.), *Handbook of the Psychology of Aging.* New York: Van Nostrand Reinhold, 1977.

Quinn, J., Segal, J., Raisz, H., and Johnson, C. (eds.) *Coordinating Community Services for the Elderly.* New York: Springer, 1982.

Redick, R. W., Kramer, M., and Taube, C. A. "Epidemiology of Mental Illness and Utilization of Psychiatric Facilities among Older Persons," in E. W. Busse and E. Pfeiffer (eds.), *Mental Illness in Later Life*. Washington, D.C.: American Psychiatric Association, 1973.

Rubenstein, L. Z., Rhee, L., and Kane, R. L. "The Role of Geriatric Assessment Units in Caring for the Elderly: An Analytic Review." *Journal of Gerontology*, 1982, *37*, 513-521.

Rucklin, H. S., Morris, J. N., and Eggert, G. M. "Management and Financing of Long Term Care Services: A New Approach to a Chronic Problem." *New England Journal of Medicine*, January 1982, *306*(2), 101.

Scanlon, W., Difederico, E., and Stassen, M. *Long-Term Care: Current Experience and a Framework for Analysis*. Washington, D.C.: The Urban Institute, 1979.

Schneider, D. "Patient/Client Assessment in New York State," in *Vol. I: Historical Review, Purposes/Uses, Framework/Recommendations*. Troy, New York: Rensselaer Polytechnic Institute, May 1980.

Skelle, F. A., Mobley, G. M., and Coan, R. E. "Cost-Effectiveness of Community-Based Long Term Care: Current Findings of Georgia's Alternative Health Services Project." *American Journal of Public Health*, 1982, *72*, 353-358.

Snider, E. L. "The Needs of Health and Related Communities Agencies Serving Elderly Families." *Canadian Journal of Public Health*, March/April 1982, *73*, 119-122.

Somers, A. R. "Long Term Care for the Elderly and Disabled: A New Health Priority." *New England Journal of Medicine*, 1982, *307*, 221-226.

Somers, A. R. "Sounding Boards: Moderating the Rise in Health-Care Costs, A programmatic Beginning." *New England Journal of Medicine*, October 1982, 944-947.

Southeast Queens Consortium of Aging Services. *Interagency Case Management Project*, Final Report, April 14, 1982.

SRI International. *Feasibility and Cost-Effectiveness of Alternative Long-Term Care Settings*. May 1978.

State Communities Association. Report of Arden House Institute on Continuity of Long Term Care. Harriman, N.Y., December, 18-20, 1977.

Steers, R. M. *Organizational Effectiveness: A Behavioral View*. Santa Monica, California: Goodyear, 1977.

Trends in Mental Health Services Coordination, Project Share: A National Clearinghouse for Improving the Management of Human Services, P.O. Box 2309, Rockville, Maryland.

Triage. *Coordinated Delivery of Services to the Elderly*, Final Report, December 1979.

Triage II. *Coordinated Delivery of Services to the Elderly*, Final Report, Vols. 1, 2 and 3, February 1982.

Vladeck, B. "Understanding Long Term Care." *New England Journal of Medicine*, September 1980, *307*, 890.

Vladeck, B. C. *Unloving Care: The Nursing Home Tragedy*. New York: Basic Books, 1980.

Weissert, W. G., Wan, T. H., Livieratos, B. and Pelligrino, J. "Cost Effectiveness of Homemaker Services for the Chronically Ill." *Inquiry*, Fall 1980, *17*, 230-243.

Weissert, W. G., Wan, T. H., Livieratos, B., and Katz, S. "Cost Effectiveness of Day Care Services for the Chronically Ill: A Randomized Experiment." *Medical Care*, June 1980, *18*(6), 567-584.

Williams, T. F., Hill, J. G., Fairbank, M. F., and Knox, K. G. "Appropriate Placement of the Chronically Ill and Aged: A Successful Approach by Evaluation." *Journal of the American Medical Association*, 1973, *226*, 1332.

Williams, M. E. and Williams, T. F. "Clinical Conference: Assessment of the Elderly for Long Term Care." *Journal of the American Geriatrics Society*, 1982, *30*(1), 71-75.

Williams, T. F. "Assessment of the Geriatric Patient in Relation to Needs for Services and Facilities," in W. Reichel, ed., *Clinical Aspects of Aging*, Second Edition. Baltimore: Williams and Wilkins, 1983.

Conference Sponsors, Speakers and Workshop Leaders

Miriam Aronson
Director
Long Term Care Gerontology Center
Einstein College of Medicine
1300 Morris Park Avenue
Bronx, New York 10104

Vicki Ashton
Center for Geriatrics and Gerontology
Columbia University
100 Haven Avenue
New York, New York 10032

Msgr. John Barry
Assistant Director
Fordham University Gerontology Center
113 West 60th Street
New York, New York 10023

Ruth Bennett
Deputy Director
Center for Geriatrics and Gerontology
Columbia University
100 Haven Avenue
New York, New York 10032

Maryann Bolles
Executive Director
Coordinated Care Management
  Corporation
237 Main Street, Room 1130
Buffalo, New York 14203

Roberta Brill
Director
Home Care Project
New York City Department for the
  Aging
280 Broadway, Room 213
New York, New York 10007

Belinda Brodows
Monroe County Long Term Care
  Program, Inc.
ACCESS
55 Troup Street
Rochester, New York 14618

Gerald Eggert
Executive Director
Monroe County Long Term Care
  Program, Inc.
55 Troup Street
Rochester, New York 14618

Msgr. Charles Fahey
Director
Third Age Center
Fordham University
113 West 60th Street
New York, New York 10023

Bill Gould
Associate Director
Jamaica Service Program for
  Older Adults
163-18 Jamaica Avenue
Jamaica, New York 11432

Goldie Green
Research Consultant
Brookdale Institute on Aging
540 West 113th Street, Apt. 3R
New York, New York 10025

Barry Gurland
Director
Center for Geriatrics and Gerontology
Columbia University
100 Haven Avenue, Tower 3-29F
New York, New York 10032

Douglas Holmes
President
Community Research Applications, Inc.
1560 Broadway, Suite 1214
New York, New York 10036

Lenard Kaye
Coordinator
Brookdale Institute on Aging
Columbia University
622 West 113th Street
New York, New York 10025

Dennis Kodner
Director
Planning and Community Services
Metropolitan Jewish Geriatric Center
4915 Tenth Avenue
Brooklyn, New York 11219

Mary Ann Lewis
Center on Gerontology
Fordham University
113 West 60th Street
New York, New York 10023

Rochelle Lipkowitz
Clinical Nurse Specialist
Long Term Care Gerontology Center
Einstein College of Medicine
1300 Morris Park Avenue
Bronx, New York 10461

Leonard McNally
Long Term Care Planner
Health Systems Agency of
   New York City
111 Broadway, 15th Floor
New York, New York 10006

Bill Mossey
Director
New York State Long Term Home
Health Care Program
40 North Pearl Street
Albany, New York 12243

Robert O'Connell
Deputy Director
Program Development and Evaluation
New York State Office for the Aged
Empire State Plaza
Albany, New York 12223

Marilyn Pickett-Desmond
New York State Health Planning
   Commission
Empire State Plaza, Tower Building,
   Room 1683
Albany, New York 12237

Alice Watson
Executive Director
Jamaica Service Program for
   Older Adults
163-18 Jamaica Avenue
Jamaica, New York 11432

David Wilder
Deputy Director
Center for Geriatrics and Gerontology
Columbia University
100 Haven Avenue
New York, New York 10032

Thomas Yandeau
Coordinator of Aging Services
Rensselaer County Department
   for the Aging
County Office Building
Troy, New York 12180

Conference Participants

Marcia Abramson
Assistant Professor
Columbia University
  School of Social Work
622 West 113th Street
New York, New York 10025

Virginia Barrett
Center for Geriatrics and Gerontology
Columbia University
100 Haven Avenue, Tower 3-29F
New York, New York 10032

Babette Becker
Executive Director
Coalition for Improved Long Term Care
c/o State Community Aid Association
23 Elk Street
Albany, New York 12207

Sharman Blake
Jamaica Service Program
  for Older Adults
163-18 Jamaica Avenue
Jamaica, New York 11432

Sarah Craig
Assistant Deputy Administrator
Long Term Care/Medical Assistant
  Program
330 West 34th Street
New York, New York 10001

Rosina Dapello
Director of Patient Services
Metropolitan Jewish Geriatric Center
West 29th Street & Boardwalk
Brooklyn, New York 11224

Joseph DeCuzzi
Director
Social Services
Amsterdam House
1060 Amsterdam Avenue
New York, New York 10025

Anne Dill
Research Associate
Brookdale Institute on Aging
  and Adult Human Development
Columbia University
622 West 113th Street
New York, New York 10025

John Dono
Research Associate
New York City Department
  for the Aging
Home Care Project
280 Broadway
New York, New York 10007

Camilla Flemming
Project FOCUS
New York City–Human Resources
  Administration
60 Hudson Street, 9th Floor
New York, New York 10013

Pat Fredericks
Director
West Side Senior Service Network
One-Stop Center
2693 Broadway
New York, New York 10025

Doris Gilman
Lennox Hill Neighborhood Association
Project SCOPE
331 East 70th Street
New York, New York 10021

Herb Golden
Jewish Home and Hospital for the Aged
120 West 106th Street
New York, New York 10025

David Gould
Project Director
Community Health and Employment
  Program
City Planning Office
2 Lafayette Street, Room 2222
New York, New York 10007

Lois Grau
Assistant Professor
School of Public Health
Columbia University
600 West 168th Street
New York, New York 10032

Richard Greenspan
New York City Department
  for the Aging
280 Broadway
New York, New York 10007

Gerta Gruen
Center for Geriatrics and Gerontology
Columbia University
100 Haven Avenue, Tower 3-29F
New York, New York 10032

Helen Hamlin
Director
Social Service Department
Metropolitan Jewish Geriatric Center
4915 Tenth Avenue
Brooklyn, New York 11219

Ellen Harnett
St. Vincent's Hospital
Long Term Care Home Health Care
  Program
153 West 11th Street
New York, New York 10011

Monica Holmes
Senior Research Associate
Community Research
1560 Broadway
New York, New York 10036

Cassandra Howard
Assistant Director/Borough Supervisor
Ombudsman Program
Community Council of Greater
  New York
225 Park Avenue South
New York, New York 10003

Jerry Joffe
New York City Department
  for the Aging
Home Care Demonstration Program
280 Broadway
New York, New York 10007

Eloise Killeffer
Research Scientist
Center for Geriatrics and Gerontology
Columbia University
100 Haven Avenue, Tower 3-29F
New York, New York 10032

Rosanne Levitt
Supervisor
Family and Adult Services
Human Resources Administration
60 Hudson Street, 9th Floor
New York, New York 10013

Betsy Mayer
Lennox Hill Neighborhood Association
Project SCOPE
331 East 70th Street
New York, New York 10021

Friedhile Milburn
Director
Network Project
New York City Department
  for the Aging
2 Lafayette Street
New York, New York 10007

Robin Mreizs
Family and Adult Services
Human Resources Administration
250 Church Street
New York, New York

Gregory Muraskiewicz
Assistant Advocate
Office of State Advocate
  for the Disabled
2 World Trade Center, Room 3712
New York, New York 10047

Anne McCarthy
Family Home Care Services
67-25 4th Avenue
Brooklyn, New York 11220

Marilyn Raymond
Director, Home Care Program
Montefiore Hospital and Medical Center
111 East 210th Street
Bronx, New York 10467

Rev. Vincent Richie
Program Officer
Center on Gerontology
Fordham University
113 West 60th Street
New York, New York 10023

Alfred Roberts
Division of Medical Assistance
New York State Department
of Social Services
40 North Pearl Street
Albany, New York 12243

Chris Rosenthal
Center on Gerontology
Fordham University
113 West 60th Street
New York, New York 10023

Vic Rosenthal
Executive Director
Coalition of Institutionalized Aged
and Disabled
Beth Abraham Hospital
612 Allerton Avenue
Bronx, New York 10467

Margareta Schaub
Supervisor
Brooklyn VNA
138 South Oxford Street
Brooklyn, New York 11217

Margaret Shannon
Center for Geriatrics and Gerontology
Columbia University
100 Haven Avenue, Tower 3-29F
New York, New York 10032

Lila Sherlock
Home Care Program
Montefiore Hospital and Medical Center
111 East 210th Street
Bronx, New York 10467

Jeanne Teresi
Senior Research Associate
Center for Geriatrics and Gerontology
Columbia University
100 Haven Avenue, Tower 3-29F
New York, New York 10032

Annie Warren
Human Resources Administration-
Family and Adult Services
60 Hudson Street
New York, New York 10013

Sophie Weiner
Borough Director
Jewish Association for Services
for the Aged
2488 Grand Concourse
Bronx, New York 10458

Robert Weiss
Dean
School of Public Health
Columbia University
600 West 168th Street
New York, New York 10032

Mel Weinstein
Home Care Project
NYC Department for the Aging
280 Broadway, Room 213
New York, New York 10007

Jane Williams
New York City Department of Health
Public Health Services
125 Worth Street, Room 203E
Box 37
New York, New York 10013

Susan Wilt
Center for Geriatrics and Gerontology
Columbia University
100 Haven Avenue, Tower 3-29F
New York, New York 10032

Stephen Wotman
Assistant Dean for Academic Affairs
School of Public Health
Columbia University
600 West 168th Street
New York, New York 10032

Marcia Wolfson
Jamaica Service Program
for Older Adults
163-18 Jamaica Avenue
Jamaica, New York 11432

Chana Zlotnik
Director
Comprehensive Family Care Center
1175 Morris Park Avenue
Bronx, New York 10104